100 Questions & Answers
About Breast Surgery

Joseph J. Disa, MD, FACS
Associate Attending Surgeon
Plastic and Reconstructive Surgery Service
Memorial Sloan-Kettering Cancer Center
New York, New York

Marie Czenko Kuechel, MA
Founder and President
Czenko Kuechel Consulting, Ltd.

D1332659

JONES AND BARTLETT PUBLISHERS
Sudbury, Massachusetts
BOSTON   TORONTO   LONDON   SINGAPORE

World Headquarters

Jones and Bartlett
Publishers
40 Tall Pine Drive
Sudbury, MA 01776
info@jbpub.com
www.jbpub.com

Jones and Bartlett
Publishers Canada
6339 Ormindale Way
Mississauga, Ontario L5V1J2
CANADA

Jones and Bartlett
Publishers International
Barb House, Barb Mews
London W6 7PA
UK

Jones and Bartlett's books and products are available through most bookstores and online book-sellers. To contact Jones and Bartlett Publishers directly, call 800-832-0034, fax 978-443-8000, or visit our website www.jbpub.com.

Substantial discounts on bulk quantities of Jones and Bartlett's publications are available to corpora-tions, professional associations, and other qualified organizations. For details and specific discount information, contact the special sales department at Jones and Bartlett via the above contact infor-mation or send an email to *specialsales@jbpub.com*.

Copyright © 2006 by Jones and Bartlett Publishers, Inc.

Library of Congress Cataloging-in-Publication Data
Disa, Joseph J.
100 questions and answers about breast surgery / Joseph J. Disa, Marie Czenko Kuechel.— 1st ed.
p. cm.
ISBN 0-7637-3041-6 (pbk.)
1. Breast—Surgery—Popular works. I. Title: One hundred questions and answers about breast surgery. II. Kuechel, Marie Czenko. III. Title.
RD539.8.D57 2006
618.1'9059—dc22
2005009008

Production Credits
Executive Publisher: Christopher Davis
Production Director: Amy Rose
Production Assistant: Kate Hennessy
Editorial Assistant: Kathy Richardson
Marketing Manager: Laura Kavigian
Manufacturing Buyer: Therese Connell
Composition: Northeast Compositors, Inc.
Cover Design: Colleen Halloran
Senior Photo Researcher: Kimberly Potvin
Cover Images: Clockwise from top left © AbleStock, © Ablestock, © Ablestock, © LiquidLibrary
Printing and Binding: Malloy, Inc.
Cover Printing: Malloy, Inc.

Printed in the United States of America
09 08 07 06 05   10 9 8 7 6 5 4 3 2 1

Dedication

This book is dedicated to my family, patients, and teachers.
Without them this would not have been possible.
Joseph J. Disa, MD, FACS

To my dear Aunt Ann Marie, a woman whose love never stops giving, to Katherine M. Marcyniuk, a friend, teacher and true hero to
the countless who love her, and to all the women who face or
choose breast surgery with the courage, faith, and passion for life
and for their future.
Marie Czenko Kuechel, MA

Contents

Part 1: Breast Surgery   1

Questions 1–6 define what breast surgery is and how it alters the appearance of the breast, including:

- What is breast surgery?
- In what ways does plastic surgery change the appearance of the breast?
- Why is breast surgery performed?

Part 2: Where to Begin   13

Questions 7–16 discuss who performs breast surgery and what factors should be considered when selecting a physician, including:

- Who performs breast surgery?
- Are these the only credentials to consider when choosing a doctor?
- Are there other factors to consider evaluating a physician?

Part 3: Breast Surgery and Safety   35

Questions 17–25 explain where breast surgery is performed and addresses patient safety concerns, including:

- Where is breast surgery performed?
- What is accreditation and why is it important?
- What are the risks of breast surgery?

Part 4: Breast Implants   49

Questions 26–39 define what breast implants are and how they are used, including:

- What are breast implants?
- When are breast implants used?
- What types of breast implants are commonly used?

Let me begin by saying it is a pleasure for me to write a foreword to this book by Joseph Disa and Maria Czenko Kuechel on *100 Questions & Answers About Breast Surgery*. Having read the draft manuscript of the book, I can say that this is quite a unique undertaking. Dr. Disa and Ms. Kuechel have written a patient- and women-friendly book on all aspects of breast surgery including cosmetic as well as reconstructive. This book is both informative and scientifically accurate about various issues associated with breast surgery, including how to choose what surgery to have as well as how to recover from or prepare for surgery.

I expect that this book will prove to be very popular to both future patients for breast surgery as well as physicians who are involved in breast surgery. I personally plan to have several copies of this book handy in my office to share with patients so that they can be more comfortable and better informed regarding breast operations.

Let me finish by congratulating Dr. Disa and Ms. Kuechel on a most informative and valuable book that should be very helpful to women who confront these issues.

Scott Spear, MD
Professor and Chief of Plastic Surgery
Department of Surgery
Georgetown University Hospital

I had the opportunity to work with Marie Kuechel on a patient information brochure regarding breast reconstruction that was published by the American Society of Plastic Surgeons. When I saw the quality of her work and dedication to accurate patient information, I eagerly accepted the offer to co-author *100 Questions & Answers About Breast Surgery*.

After completing my undergraduate education at the University of Notre Dame, and medical education at the University of Massachusetts Medical School, I completed two residencies. The first was in general surgery at the University of Maryland Medical Systems and the second in Plastic and Reconstructive Surgery at the Johns Hopkins/University of Maryland Hospitals. I completed my post-graduate education in Plastic Surgery by doing a reconstructive microsurgery fellowship at the Memorial Sloan-Kettering Cancer Center. Upon the completion of my fellowship, I became part of the full-time faculty at Memorial Sloan-Kettering Cancer Center. Currently, as a board-certified plastic surgeon and member of the American Society of Plastic Surgeons, I practice at Sloan-Kettering and contribute to the education of students, surgeons in training, and practicing surgeons nationally and internationally.

Memorial Sloan-Kettering Cancer Center is a major provider for cancer and allied disease in the greater New York area, with a patient base that spans the globe. My practice has evolved into one dominated by aesthetic and reconstructive breast surgery. The approach at our institution to the management of breast disease is multidisciplinary, and involves medical, surgical, and radiation oncologists, radiologists, pathologists, psychiatrists, and plastic surgeons. Therefore, the opportunity to reach out from my normal practice of individualized patient education prior to mandatory or elective breast surgery, and contribute to this book was a terrific opportunity.

The era of the Internet, and the plethora of both visual and print media regarding breast surgery can be overwhelming. A Web search of breast surgery (both elective and non-elective) will provide a mountain of information that can be as unreliable and misleading as it is educational. Similarly, sensationalized television programming regarding plastic surgery can be equally misleading. The availability of information has allowed patients to become more sophisticated regarding their health care and the choices available to them. Patients who are more educated will have more confidence about the process they are contemplating or undergoing, which can help to manage expectations. However, as important as information and education are, misinformation can be detrimental. The opportunity to provide sound education and dispel the myths regarding the most common questions that arise when considering breast surgery is the premise of this book.

Joseph J. Disa, MD, FACS

Early in my career, at age 24, I was developing patient education on plastic surgery procedures for the American Society of Plastic Surgeons. It was a time when what was labeled "The Breast Implant Crisis" had come to a peak. A lot of what I learned at that time, and the people from whom I learned, influenced both my career and me as a person.

I learned that in the world there were talented, passionate, compassionate surgeons who performed breast procedures to fulfill the lives of women. I learned that, conversely, there were imposters whose only fulfillment was their own pocket. I learned that the media was a powerful machine that could set agendas and build you up high. Conversely, I learned the media was just as powerful at bringing you down, once there was no longer a story on which to build you higher. And, I learned that my soon-to-be aunt-by-marriage, Anne Marie, full of the most genuine passion for life, was diagnosed with breast cancer.

Today the focus of my work is somewhat broader: it includes physicians, medical societies, pharmaceutical companies, and medical device manufacturers. But the goal I define as my life's work remains the same as it was in those early days. My work must benefit patients—the consumers of medicine. And, equally important, my work must uphold and enrich the ability of the passionate, talented surgeons, men and women who continue to inspire me with dedication to their patients and profession, to communicate with and educate their patients.

One would think that it is tough for me to remain focused on my goals, given the constant and growing influence of media and influx of providers who give breast surgery and plastic surgery a very bad image. Rather, these things drive me to make certain that my work remains focused and has value. Before I had even completed the writing of the book, *100 Questions & Answers About Plastic Surgery* with Diane L. Gerber, MD (published by Jones and Bartlett Publishers in 2004), I set out to write this book. I believed that a single book about plastic surgery could not answer all of a woman's questions about breast surgery. I believed that it required 100 questions of its own.

Aunt Anne Marie did not live long enough to consider breast reconstruction. But, today, many more women do survive than only a decade ago. These women who undergo breast surgery to treat or prevent disease or to reconstruct a breast lost or disfigured by breast disease deserve thorough and candid information to learn about their options, find a qualified provider, and make a confident decision. This is equally true for women who elect to have breast surgery to improve the size, shape, or position of their breasts.

I hope this book provides all of the unbiased information you need about breast surgery, and that it guides you to choosing a qualified provider. Through reading these questions and answers, and with the support of those who love you, I know you can make a decision that is right and fulfilling for you.

Marie Czenko Kuechel, MA

One of the greatest things about being a physician is the ability to interact in a meaningful and personal way with so many different people. As a plastic surgeon, particularly working at a cancer hospital, I have the opportunity to provide hope for people facing physical disfigurement from their disease. The amount of courage and strength that I see day after day in my patients, their friends, and families is awe-inspiring. I am incredibly grateful and thankful for the ability to meet these people, participate in their care, and hopefully impact their lives in a positive way.

Part of being a physician involves a significant amount of time away from home and unending support from one's family. It is rarely possible to completely separate yourself from your practice and therefore it is always part of your life. I am fortunate to have a loving and supportive family. To my wife, Julie, who has been there through medical school, two residencies, a fellowship, and many years of practice, you have always been the voice of reason, and unconditionally supportive...I can't begin to thank you enough. To Michael and Nicholas, who with their smiles and amazing personalities make every day a bright one, I thank you both very much.

I would like to thank Marie Kuechel for involving me in this project and Jones and Bartlett Publishers for recognizing the need for this book. This book covers an extremely important topic and has the opportunity to be a vital resource for women contemplating breast surgery. It is an honor to be a part of this project.

Joseph J. Disa, MD, FACS

I believe in giving thanks, every day. Each day of life is something to be thankful for, and gives hope for the days to come. Upon this, my third book, my thanks grow stronger and reach wider than ever before.

To all the women and men who face their challenges and choices in life with confidence, education, and the courage to forge ahead—thank you for your inspiration. To all of the women facing or choosing breast surgery whom I have known, read about, or who may have benefited from any one of the educational endeavors I have contributed to, thank you for adding purpose to my profession.

Professionally, there is a world of amazing providers in medicine who I thank for their integrity and dedication to their specialties and patients. Most notably, from the earliest days of my career through to today, I am grateful for the leadership, patience, and kindness of: James H. Wells, MD, James G. Hoehn, MD, Mark L. Jewell, MD, Foad Nahai, MD, Walter E. Erhardt, MD, Brian Kinney, MD, and Diane L. Gerber, MD. Thank you to Scott L. Spear, MD for his support and contributions to this project. To Robert Singer, MD and Simon Fredricks, MD, thank you for treating me with the respect of a peer—your trust and support of my work and my drive is something that makes me immensely grateful and proud.

Some would find it amazing that upon an email and a few short exchanges, my co-author Joe Disa, MD agreed to this book. But the instant you meet him, his genuinely kind and dedicated nature shines. Add to this his research and work in advancing breast reconstruction and all breast surgeries, and there is no question that his role as a co-author is most appropriate. Thank you, Joe, for helping me to make this very important project a reality.

Professionally, I have many friends who deserve my thanks, too: Bob Stanton and his amazing team at the American Society for Aesthetic Plastic Surgery, the dedicated staff of the American Society of Plastic Surgeons, and all of my clients and their kind staff who are more like family and friends than business acquaintances. Thanks to the coach who has taken me through some stressful times and helped me to find what is beginning to resemble a tennis game, Michael Byrd. And, many thanks to Mark Liss, Esq., for his patience, guidance, and amazing listening.

The patience, support, and love of family are something that people live to expect and something I have never taken for granted.

To my parents, Victor and Maria, you expected nothing less than I do my best in life. Thank you for setting the bar high and for helping me to reach it. To you, my godmother Helen, in-laws Theresa and Andreas, and our housekeeper Teresa, thank you for all of your support, time babysitting, and amazing listening skills.

To John, Nicholas, and Andrew, you expect nothing more of me, than to love you. And you know that with all I am and all I do, there is nothing more in the world I love than the three of you. Nicky and Andy—never did I think I would author three books in two years, much less a lifetime; never did I think I would have two such amazing children who also can accomplish anything you expect of yourself.

Marie Czenko Kuechel, MA

Breast Surgery: Diversity, Disease, and Desire

The single most visible feature that defines a woman's appearance is the presence of breasts. And while many women choose not to define themselves by their breasts, to many women breast size, position, shape, and health is a very defining issue.

Breast surgery is as diverse in procedures and outcomes as women are in appearance: from reducing large breasts, to enhancing small breasts, to lifting sagging breasts; from removing diseased breast tissue to then restoring a breast disfigured by or lost to disease. However, breast surgery involves much more than the physical outcomes that result to a woman's figure. Breast surgery is highly emotional: when elected to enhance appearance it is highly fulfilling. When prescribed to treat disease, it may be both devastating to lose a breast, yet rewarding to be cured, and even more rewarding to be restored through reconstruction.

A woman's breasts are the most visible and consistent symbol that define her as a physical person, and that define women in the eyes of industry, far beyond simply the medical industry. Consider these facts about commerce and industry driven by and supporting women's breast and health issues, and the influence of media attention on what is a highly intimate, yet very public issue:

- In 2004, the American Society of Plastic Surgeons reported that 445,438 women underwent surgery to enlarge, lift, or reduce breast size. The collective fees for these procedures based on data from the American Society of Aesthetic Plastic Surgery, was $2.342 million.
- In 2003, the largest manufacturer and retailer of lingerie, Victoria's Secret, had net retail sales of $2,822 million, of which the Miracle Bra®, Water Bra®, and Second Skin Satin® were their

highest sellers. The Japanese-based company, Wacoal, was the second leading bra manufacturer, with wholesale sales of $1,386.5 million in 2003.

- In 1992, in what was titled a "Breast Implant Crisis," silicone gel-filled breast implants were recalled for use in breast augmentation by the U.S. Food and Drug Administration (FDA) for suspicion that they contributed to auto-immune diseases in some women. Later, independent reports by the National Institutes of Health refuted those claims, and then-U.S. Surgeon General C. Everett Koop, MD, called the entire event "a great fraud" perpetuated on American women by the media.

- Breast reduction is a growing procedure among women, despite the ebb and flow in coverage by the insurance industry for a procedure proven in clinical studies (BRAVO: Breast Reduction Assessment and Value of Outcomes study) to improve a woman's mobility, decrease physical pain and disability, and enhance her overall quality of life and health, and despite new research that indicates breast reduction, in some cases, can reduce a woman's chance of developing breast cancer by 50% to 70%.

- Current data show breast cancer cures on the rise, and breast reconstruction surgeries on the decline. But the picture is incomplete because those statistics include the newest surgical innovations that don't necessarily require reconstruction—innovations that conserve breast tissue and, thus, in many cases retain the presence of a woman's breast.

- American industry has become actively involved in supporting issues related to women and their breasts. The cosmetics company Avon sponsors the Walk for the Cure; the pink ribbon campaign was invented in 1991 by Evelyn H. Lauder, founder and president of Estee Lauder Cosmetics as the symbol for breast cancer awareness, of which automakers from BMW to Ford have been visible sponsors. American icon Ralph Lauren designed the "Pink Pony" campaign to fund a breast center for underserved communities in conjunction with New York's Memorial Sloan-Kettering Cancer Center. Even the United

States Postal Service initiated a pink ribbon postage stamp from which the additional postage collected is donated to breast cancer research.

No one judges a woman by her Wonderbra® nor ridicules her for the need to lift, separate, and minimize. No one questions industry's use of breast cancer awareness to publicize themselves. But we question the use of implants, cringe at the thought of removing healthy breast tissue, and even debate why a woman would restore a breast following mastectomy rather than be thankful for life and simply wear a prosthesis. If the presence, appearance, size, and shape of a woman's breast were not important to her, then breast surgery would not exist except for treating disease. But, then neither would the plethora of lingerie, devices, herbs, creams, and potions designed with the intent to somehow improve or enhance a woman's breasts.

Women have questions. Women want answers. But where can they turn in the mass of media, marketing, and mayhem? This book is where any woman and those who support her, love her, and question her desire for breast surgery can turn for candid answers to the questions women have, and deserve to have answered about breast surgery.

Except in the case of disease, the question most often asked of any breast surgery is, why? Why undergo surgery electively, on something that can be padded or uplifted so easily, or reduced with industrial strength fibers, so simply? The answer is that, to many women, the ability to look at one's self image and feel wholly fulfilled, and the freedom and confidence to wear what they want, when they want, and move about as freely as they want, is an immensely satisfying experience that is well worth the physical, emotional, and financial costs associated with breast surgery.

The questions in this book include some of the answers about cost, but don't attach monetary cost to any procedure. Monetary costs can only be determined when the course of treatment is defined. But cost of any kind is fundamental to understanding, and accepting the desire or the need, the possibilities, and the process of breast surgery. And while this book offers the answers to 100 questions about breast surgery, each woman considering or facing breast surgery likely has countless more questions of her own. That is why choosing someone to perform your breast surgery is as thoroughly discussed as the procedures themselves. Use this guide to choose someone who can answer your individual questions. But don't stop there.

Use this guide to evaluate your surgeon, your safety, and your own motivations for breast surgery. But make the decision to have breast surgery yours alone. While others may influence you, support you, or deter you, it is only the woman who chooses to undergo breast surgery who must live with her decision, the experience, and the outcomes that decision brings. And the outcomes, indeed, can be very fulfilling.

PART ONE

Breast Surgery

What is breast surgery?

In what ways does plastic surgery change
the appearance of the breast?

Why is breast surgery performed?

More...

1. What is breast surgery?

Breast surgery is defined as any medical procedure that penetrates beyond the surface of breast skin. Breast surgery ranges from procedures as limited as a needle biopsy, to something as complex as microsurgical post-mastectomy breast reconstruction.

Breast surgery can be defined in two broad categories:

- Procedures to diagnose and treat breast disease including cancer and benign cysts, tumors, and growths
- Procedures to change the appearance of a breast, including restoring the absence of a breast, increase or decrease in breast size, or revision of breast shape and position

Recently, however, a third category of breast surgery has emerged: surgery to prevent breast disease. While prophylactic **bilateral mastectomy** has been elected as early as the 1980s to significantly reduce a woman's chances for developing breast cancer, it only recently has become an accepted practice in the prevention of breast disease in women who are carriers of the breast cancer genes *BRCA1 and BRCA2*. Studies show that there is a 90% reduction in the incidence of breast cancer among these women. However, recent studies have demonstrated that even women who are not carriers of the breast cancer gene can, in fact, reduce their chances of developing breast cancer. In a study published in the June 2004 issue of *Plastic and Reconstructive Surgery*, women with overly large breasts and without the presence of certain genetic factors relative to breast cancer who underwent breast reduction were found to have a reported 50% to 70% reduction in the incidence of

Breast surgery

any medical procedure that penetrates beyond the surface of breast skin. Includes: (1) procedures to diagnose and treat breast disease including cancer and benign cysts, tumors, and growths; (2) procedures to change the appearance of a breast, including restoring the absence of a breast, increase or decrease in breast size, or revision of breast shape and position; and (3) surgery to prevent breast disease.

Bilateral mastectomy

surgical removal of both breasts.

BRCA1 and BRCA2

genes found to be linked to a predisposition for breast cancer.

breast cancer. (These two examples are discussed in depth in Questions 48 and 72, respectively.)

Beyond the categories of breast surgery to either treat disease or change appearance, breast surgery can also be defined by medical specialty:

- **General breast surgery**: to diagnose and treat breast disease through the removal of the entire breast, or only of diseased tissue, tumors, or cysts
- **Plastic surgery of the breast**: any surgical procedure that changes or restores the appearance of the breast, including those procedures to treat and prevent breast disease that result in the change of breast appearance

2. In what ways does plastic surgery change the appearance of the breast?

Plastic surgery of the breast can change breast appearance by:

- Making large breasts smaller (**breast reduction**)
- Making small breasts larger (**breast augmentation**)
- Restoring the appearance of a sagging, flat breast (**breast lift**)
- Restoring the appearance of a breast disfigured or removed by disease (**breast reconstruction**)
- Restoring symmetry to the appearance of the breasts following surgery to treat disease or reconstruct a breast (all of the above)
- Restoring a more normal appearance to breast anomalies or congenital (from birth) and developmental deformities: misshapen or tubular breasts, breasts that develop disproportionately, and correc-

General breast surgery

to diagnose and treat breast disease through the removal of the entire breast, or only of diseased tissue, tumors, or cysts.

Plastic surgery for breast reconstruction

a specialty of medicine that includes board-certified training specific to the techniques and procedures that rebuild a breast mound including the nipple and areola.

Breast reduction

a type of surgery that removes fat and/or glandular tissue to reduce size and reshape a woman's breasts.

Breast augmentation

procedure to make small breasts larger.

Breast lift

procedure to restore the appearance of a sagging, flat breast.

Breast reconstruction

restoring the appearance of a breast disfigured or removed by disease.

Breast Surgery

tion of rare conditions such as the presence of more than one nipple on the breast
- Treating breast disease while preserving the most normal appearance of the breast; this includes the removal of cysts and tumors, breast conserving surgery, skin sparring mastectomy, and mastectomy

Although plastic surgery can change the appearance of the breast in many different ways, based on the many different cases that present, the goal for plastic surgery of the breast is always to restore or retain a normal appearance. In some cases, a more normal appearance simply means bringing balance to a woman's figure. In others it requires complete reconstruction of a breast and surgery to alter the appearance of the opposite breast to match the size and position of the breast that is reconstructed.

Yet while plastic surgery of the breast may have one common goal for all women, it remains a highly individualized procedure based on:

- A woman's preferences and perceptions for her body
- A woman's physical anatomy and her figure
- A woman's overall health and prognosis
- The recommendations of a qualified board-certified plastic surgeon

As much as these factors influence what plastic surgery of the breast can achieve for a woman, they equally are limitations to what, in some cases, plastic surgery of the breast may *not* be able to achieve. For example, while breast reconstruction can create a very natural appearing breast in which a woman may have some sensation, in no way can plastic surgery of the breast create a breast to exactly replace one in appearance, function, and sensation that is lost or disfigured by surgery, disease, or even accidental trauma.

Consider, too, that there are limitations for a woman who desires to increase breast size so significantly that her present skin cannot possibly stretch to accommodate the size of the implant. Equally, there may be limitations for a woman with enormous breasts who wishes to retain the ability to breast-feed after reduction. Despite modern techniques that retain the function and sensation of the nipple, if a woman's breast size is primarily mammary tissue, reduction will, in fact, affect a woman's ability to breast-feed.

Plastic surgery of the breast can make a remarkable difference in the appearance of a woman's breast, in the way a woman sees herself, and in the way others see her. But women must approach what plastic surgery of the breast can achieve with realistic expectations: plastic surgery of the breast can improve the appearance of a woman's breast and her figure as a whole, but it cannot achieve perfection. Based on a woman's current physical condition and what it will take to achieve realistic goals, there are always trade-offs. These trade-offs, however, are well worth it for the over one half million women who undergo plastic surgery of the breast each year in the United States.*

---

*Compiled from the American Society of Plastic Surgeons annual report on plastic surgery procedures, 2003, including only breast augmentation, reduction, lift, and reconstruction.

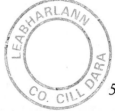

3. Why is breast surgery performed?

Breast surgery is performed for a number of reasons, not simply because a woman either needs or wants breast surgery. Breast surgery is performed because it is:

- Recommended or prescribed as the course of treatment for disease
- Recommended, prescribed, or elected to prevent disease
- Recommended or prescribed to improve a woman's physical condition and quality of life
- Desired to improve a woman's physical condition and quality of life
- Desired to bring proportion to a woman's figure
- Desired to restore changes in a woman's figure
- Desired to enhance personal appearance

In every case, breast surgery has theoretical alternatives. A woman can reject mastectomy or any form of tissue removal to treat disease despite paramount detriment to her health. Or, less aggressive forms of treatment combinations may be appropriate substitutes, such as lumpectomy with radiation or skin sparring mastectomy with immediate reconstruction. To further the alternatives, a woman can reject reconstruction altogether and wear a prosthesis, or she may even choose not to hide her condition.

A small-breasted woman may wear padded bras rather than undergo augmentation. A large-breasted woman may hide behind baggy clothing and minimizing bras to de-emphasize overly large breasts. Another woman may choose to wear a bra around the clock, and never appear unclothed even to her partner or spouse to hide deeply sagging, flat breasts. She may exercise herself to exhaustion, believing that fitness relates to the condition of her breasts. Or, a woman may purchase creams, herbal supplements, and devices with the promise of improving her breast condition.

But none of these alternatives has the same proven result as breast surgery, in any case, prescribed or elective. The proof is in the continued evolution of techniques in procedures for breast surgery, and in the satisfaction of women who have undergone breast surgery to save or change their lives.

I was always an active, athletic woman. No frills about my body; I just wanted a healthy body. I wondered why some women focused so much on their bodies, and their breasts. But the day I learned I had breast cancer, and learned that I would lose my breast, my thinking of why women were so focused on their breasts changed quickly to, "why do I have to lose mine?"

—Ann G., age 36 when diagnosed with breast cancer

4. Who has breast surgery?

Women of all ages, all races, all income, and all education levels have breast surgery. There is no one factor that defines all breast surgery patients. In fact, women are not the only breast surgery patients; men can undergo breast surgery, too.

Women who choose to undergo breast augmentation (the surgical placement of implants to enhance breast size and shape) are not only people seen in the media. In fact, most women who choose augmentation are restoring breast volume lost after pregnancy and breast-feeding. Likewise are women who elect surgery to reduce the size of overly large breasts. Most women with overly large breasts are not, in fact, obese or generally even overweight. Breast size is largely determined by heredity. So too, is how a woman's breast ages determined by heredity, not fitness. A very active and fit woman with poor skin elasticity can find that, over time, her breasts point downward and no longer outward.

Women who undergo breast surgery to treat disease are not all post-menopausal, or women who lack a healthy lifestyle. They are of every age and some are the picture of fitness and health. They are not all severely disfigured or debilitated by surgery or by the effects of disease and prescribed treatment. More often these women lead happy lives and have a positive outlook. They do not hide their condition; they share their experiences and support one another. Women who choose to reconstruct a breast lost or disfigured to breast disease are not ungrateful for their cure, but are largely grateful for the opportunity to feel whole and optimistic about leading a normal life.

Men who undergo breast surgery are those who are diagnosed with breast disease or who elect to have surgery. Elective breast surgery for men is most commonly to correct a condition called **gynecomastia** (which is the excessive growth of male mammary glands) using a type of surgery that achieves a more masculine appearance to an enlarged male breast. While the issue of breast surgery for men is an important one, it deserves

Gynecomastia

excessive development of male mammary glands.

a focus of its own, because much of women's health and men's health issues differ so greatly.

This book is not written for or about the women who have had breast surgery. Rather, it is written for any woman who is curious about, desires, or has been recommended to undergo breast surgery of any kind. It is also for the people who love, support, and believe in her.

For more general information about breast cancer and breast surgery for men and women, visit the National Library of Medicine and National Institutes of Health Medline Plus at *www.nlm.nih. gov/medlineplus.* Here you will find a general encyclopedia of information on health topics as well as recent accepted findings, statistics, and treatment innovations, and links to resources for additional information. For national statistics on plastic surgery of the breast, visit *www.plasticsurgery.org.*

5. Why would I want to undergo breast surgery?

Want and need are two very different things, and are subjective to many people. To some, need is about desire, it is not an absolute in order to survive. To others, need is what one must accept to survive. Much of the focus of this book is about want. It is about the desire to enhance or change one's breast appearance to achieve a personal goal. But want/desire in fact is attached to need in every case. Even in the case of need, a woman wants for certain outcomes.

Why you would want to undergo breast surgery is a very important question that you must ask yourself, and be able to realistically answer yourself. No one can ask or answer the question for you, nor can anyone but you make your decision.

In asking why you want to undergo breast surgery, define your goals. What is it you want to achieve for your body and for your life? The answer to why you would want to undergo breast surgery will be based on knowledge and understanding of your condition, of a given procedure, and on the recommendations of a qualified provider.

Be realistic in what you desire, that is, in what you want to achieve, and be thorough when seeking your answers. But don't stop questioning once you determine your want. Defining why you want breast surgery is only the first step to your experience with breast surgery.

Wanting to have breast surgery is something I thought about and joked about for a long time. But there came a day when accepting that I had gone from a 34C to a 34A after two pregnancies, wasn't something I could joke about anymore. I would tell any woman who wants to have breast surgery that you will think about, joke about, maybe even be embarrassed about wanting it, before you finally find someone to confide in and talk to about it. But whatever phase you are in, your answer as to why you want breast surgery will always be the same: "Because I want it!"

—Kristin M., age 39, mother of 2

6. *Where do I begin?*

You begin by defining your realistic goals, what it is you want breast surgery to achieve for you. Be specific, be realistic, and be comfortable discussing your goals.

Then discuss your goals with a qualified provider. Talk, listen, take notes, and ask questions. If you don't feel comfortable with the answers that you are given, or the provider giving the answers, seek advice from another qualified provider.

The beginning of this process may seem simplistic, but indeed it is not. There are many questions to ask, a great deal of information to evaluate, choices and decisions to face, and emotional and physical experiences to live, all in defining your goals and in determining exactly what can be achieved for you, personally. This entire experience is vital to your safety and satisfaction with breast surgery, and is detailed in Part II: Where to Begin.

Perhaps the most important aspect of successful breast surgery is to state your goals and expectations realistically, and likewise to have what can be realistically achieved through breast surgery defined to you by your provider. This is essential to avoid an unfulfilled situation where the outcomes of breast surgery do not meet your expectations.

If you have been referred for breast surgery to diagnose breast disease, or have been diagnosed with breast disease, your primary resource through your experience will be your board-certified gynecologist. According to the American College of Obstetrics and Gynecology, "training in gynecology covers women's general health, including care of reproductive organs, breasts, and sexual function. Screening for cancer at multiple sites is performed or initiated by the Ob-Gyn specialist."

While an obstetrician/gynecologist (OB/GYN) does not treat breast disease, he or she is the primary care provider of women's health and should be involved and accessible to you throughout your treatment experience. For more information on the role of a gynecologist and to find a board-certified gynecologist in your community, visit *www.acog.org.*

PART TWO

Where to Begin

Who performs breast surgery?

Are these the only credentials to consider
when choosing a doctor?

Are there other factors to consider in
evaluating a physician?

More...

7. Who performs breast surgery?

Unbelievably, breast surgery *can* be performed by any physician regardless of specialty. A physician does not have to be trained in breast surgery or plastic surgery to offer these procedures to patients. For example, any physician can purchase breast implants and place them into a woman's body, if he or she has access to the necessary equipment and facility to do so.

Unfortunately, there is currently no legislative or other legal means to restrict physicians from performing certain types of medical procedures, regardless of skill or training. As a patient, you need to know who is qualified to perform breast surgery and plastic surgery of the breast. You must take the initiative to verify and recognize adequate training, experience, board certification, and credentials that directly relate to the procedure you are considering or that has been prescribed for you. Only then can you begin to consider a physician qualified to perform your breast surgery.

Board certification

a process following the completion of medical school that includes several years of additional training in a medical specialty, written and oral exams, and continuing hours of education after certification by the American Board of Medical Specialties (ABMS) in the United States.

In general, there are two categories of board-certified physicians who perform breast surgery: plastic surgeons and general surgeons. **Board certification*** is recognized by nationally and internationally accepted standards. In the United States, the presiding organization is the American Board of Medical Specialties. It is a very complex and thorough process of training

---

*Board-eligible providers who have not yet completed written and oral exams can be considered qualified providers of breast surgery in the medical specialties defined in this book. When you consult with a provider who is not yet board certified, ask that provider when board certification is anticipated. You should also question a provider who has finished training many years previously and is not yet board-certified.

in a specialty that takes several years after graduation from medical school, and involves oral and written exams, plus hours of continuing education following certification.

In the United States, the American Board of Medical Specialties (*www.abms.org*) is the umbrella organization of 24 approved medical specialty boards, including surgery and plastic surgery. "The intent of the (ABMS) certification of physicians is to provide assurance to the public that those certified by an ABMS Member Board have successfully completed an approved training program and an evaluation process assessing their ability to provide quality patient care in the specialty." In Canada, board certification is defined and awarded by the Royal College of Physicians & Surgeons of Canada (*www.rcpsc.medical.org*).

Board-Certified Plastic Surgeons

Any surgical procedure of the breast, except those performed strictly to diagnose breast disease, is appropriately performed by a board-certified plastic surgeon. Breast augmentation, reduction, lift, and reconstruction as well as any procedure to restore or enhance the shape or appearance of the breast should only be performed by a board-certified plastic surgeon. Plastic surgery is the only medical specialty with training in accredited surgical residency specific to surgical procedures that can restore or enhance the shape of the breast.

Only one board recognized by the American Board of Medical Specialties certifies a plastic surgeon: The American Board of Plastic Surgery (*www.abplsurg.org*). Those holding ABPS certification are the only physicians to appropriately hold the title "plastic surgeon" and can perform plastic surgery of the face and entire body, including the breast. Physicians with board certification in other specialties are not accredited to perform **all** types of breast surgery, specifically plastic surgery procedures of the breast.

Board-Certified Surgeons

Qualified providers of those breast surgery procedures limited to diagnosing or treating breast disease are "general" surgeons certified by the American Board of Surgery (*www.absurgery.org*). The board defines these surgeons as having the "training, knowledge, and experience related to the diagnosis, preoperative, operative, and postoperative management, including the management of complications, in the essential content areas." Board certification in surgery includes experience and training in:

• Surgical oncology (surgery to treat cancer)
• Biopsy techniques for breast cancer
• Stereotactic breast biopsy techniques including advanced breast biopsy instrumentation (ABBI)
• Core needle biopsy and mammotome techniques
• Diagnostic ultrasonography of the breast

It is important to know that as of the publication of this book, within the specialty of surgery and among all ABMS recognized specialties, there is no recognized credential or subspecialty specific to breast surgery. There is technically no defined, recognized credential defining a "breast surgeon," except that all board-certified plastic surgeons do have accredited training and core competency in plastic surgery procedures of the breast.

Access to Information

The following Web sites offer definitions of board certification. All but the American Board of Surgery provide you with the opportunity to confirm a physician's board certification with the related specialty.

American Board of Medical Specialties: *http://www.abms.org*
Royal College of Physicians & Surgeons of Canada:
  http://www.rcpsc.medicine.org
American Board of Plastic Surgery: *http://www.abplsurg.org*
American Board of Surgery: *http://www.absurgery.org*

Action has begun at the state level to introduce legislation regarding physician advertising and medical education. In 2004, California upheld state legislation that limits physician advertising to content related to one's specialty, and limits the use of the term "board-certified" to specialties with approved by the American Board of Medical Specialties. At the same time, Florida introduced legislation that would require physicians to disclose ABMS board certification in advertising and require physicians to specify medical training. This legislation does not preclude the need for consumers to research provider credentials. But it does highlight board certification and specialization, which are the starting point of choosing a qualified provider in any medical specialty.

8. Are these the only credentials to consider when choosing a doctor?

Checking board certification is a good place to begin; however, in no way is board certification the only qualification. Beyond board certification you should consider a provider's specialized training and experience in performing a given procedure.

Furthermore, even though a procedure may be performed in a physician's office-based surgical facility or an outpatient surgical facility, you must make certain that your physician has privileges to perform that same procedure in a local, accredited hospital or full-service medical center. A physician who is on staff and has **privileges** to perform specific plastic surgery and breast surgery procedures at an accredited hospital has had his or her training and credentials reviewed by that hospital's board of medical specialists before being given privileges.

9. Are there other factors to consider in evaluating a physician?

When evaluating a board-certified plastic or general surgeon to perform your breast surgery, you should also review and consider appropriate providers of specific treatments and professional affiliations.

- Appropriate providers for procedures that are considered plastic surgery of the breast, or that will change the appearance or shape of your breast in any way are board-certified plastic surgeons. These procedures include: breast augmentation, breast reduction, breast reconstruction, breast lift, and surgery to treat anomalies and deformities. In some cases, a plastic surgeon may also perform procedures to remove breast tumors and cysts, lumpectomy, breast-conserving surgery, and procedures to remove the breast entirely including mastectomy and skin-sparing mastectomy; however, these are more commonly performed by a general surgeon. This is often done in consultation with a plastic surgeon, if reconstruction is indicated.
- Appropriate providers for procedures to diagnose or treat breast disease including biopsy, procedures to

Privileges

a type of agreement for a physician to operate in a particular accredited hospital; the doctor's credentials, knowledge, and training, medical standards in a particular specialty, and skills are rigorously examined by his or her peers before privileges are extended.

remove breast tumors and cysts, lumpectomy, breast-conserving surgery, and all forms of mastectomy are board-certified surgeons.

Among board-certified plastic surgeons and general surgeons, professional affiliations include, most specifically, the organizations that support the training, education, and research of plastic surgery or surgery in general, and of physicians holding appropriate qualifications to perform specific breast surgery procedures. In addition, these organizations require certain standards of practice, ethics, and continuing medical education, all with the mission to uphold patient safety.

Board-Certified Plastic Surgeons

For board-certified plastic surgeons, look for membership in the American Society of Plastic Surgeons (ASPS). ASPS requires members be board certified by the American Board of Plastic Surgery, and requires added ongoing training and competency in plastic surgery procedures. The organization also requires members to adhere to safety standards and ethical standards that include such things as advertising, patient rights, and privacy.

Board-certified plastic surgeons can belong to subspecialty groups. For example, those board-certified plastic surgeons practicing **aesthetic plastic surgery** (which are procedures specifically to enhance appearance) may belong to the American Society for Aesthetic Plastic Surgery (ASAPS). But the primary professional membership for any board-certified plastic surgeon is the American Society of Plastic Surgeons.

Aesthetic plastic surgery

procedures elected strictly to improve breast appearance and a woman's appearance overall.

19

Board-Certified Surgeons

The American College of Surgeons (ACS) is the professional organization of all surgical specialties, including plastic surgery and general surgery. Member surgeons are defined by specialty. Like ASPS, the ACS has membership requirements and continuing education requirements for their members as well as safety and ethical standards.

Surgeons can also belong to sub-specialty groups. The American Society of Breast Surgeons is a professional group of surgeons formed to encourage the study of breast surgery, to promote research and development of advanced surgery techniques, and to improve standards of practice for breast surgery in the United States. The Society of Surgical Oncologists is a professional group that serves surgeons who specialize in the treatment of oncologic disease.

Suddenly you are considering breast surgery, and it not as easy as one thinks to understand who is the right breast doctor for you. The medical societies are your best resource, and you can be confident that the information and resources they provide are in the public's best interests. And, many of them make it easy to review a doctor's credentials, learn something about him or her, and the procedure you want before even calling the office.

—Kristin

I agree, but when suddenly you are faced with the need for surgery, and your health and appearance are at stake, doing your homework can be very frustrating. That is why I think so many women just listen to their doctor and accept what they are told, like it or not, instead of questioning, or consulting others to understand all of their options. The emotions you feel are immensely stressful, but when you find the right doctor, you know, because that stress suddenly becomes hope.

—Ann

10. How do I find a qualified provider?

The two most common means of finding a qualified provider to perform your breast surgery include referral and your own research. Combining both of these clearly can be most effective.

You also should consider the influence of the many physicians who advertise plastic surgery of the breast. If you are considering plastic surgery of the breast, hopefully, you won't find or seek out a provider by responding to bargain advertisements or special offers. While advertising is a common and acceptable practice, it may not tell you the whole story. Always check credentials and seek out some form of referral to that physician.

Referral

A referral by a trusted physician, family member, or friend is a good first step in finding the breast or plastic surgeon who is right for you. In addition, many hospital- and university-based medical centers offer referral services. Even if your referral is from a trusted physician to treat disease, make your final selection for a provider based on your research of credentials, affiliations, and the appropriateness of treatment relative to credentials and experience.

Research

Research today most often begins on the Internet. In your Internet directory searches for a breast surgery provider, first consider the directories of the medical societies and professional organizations that support physicians qualified to perform breast surgery and plastic surgery of the breast. Most of these groups have directories or referral services available online.

Aside from these medical boards and professional societies, you need to be cautious of the sources you are using for your research. Those Web sites that pop up first on a search of "breast surgery" are not necessarily the most credible sources of information. Many directories, physician finder, and listing services available online are commonly subscription services where a physician pays to be listed, and there may be no requirement or screening of credentials. *You* must always check credentials.

Once you have carefully confirmed a provider's board certification, affiliations, training, and experience check on the licensing or accreditation of the facility where your surgery will be performed. This is thoroughly discussed in Part 3 of this book.

Physician Online Directories of Qualified Breast Surgery Providers:

The American Society of Plastic Surgeons:
www.plasticsurgery.org
The American Society for Aesthetic Plastic Surgery:
www.surgery.org
The American College of Surgeons: *www.facs.org*

---

11. What, beyond credentials, should I consider when making a decision on providers?

Credentials are your foundation and experience is your framework, yet every physician is an individual. A consultation is your opportunity to meet the individual and to ask a provider specifically how he or she will address your case. In your consultation, be sure to personally review the specific credentials of the provider you are considering, and make certain all credentials are active and in good standing. Then ask specific questions about the kind of experience the provider has relative to the procedure you are considering or that has been prescribed for you. Realize that experience is not always measured in years—it is measured in satisfied patients and in outcomes.

How you gauge experience and determine your personal comfort with a provider is by listening, by reviewing, and by asking questions. These questions may include asking the provider how many times he or she has performed the specific procedure you are considering, or that is recommended for you. Listen to how a provider speaks and what he or she says when consulting with you:

- Is he or she confident, clear, and direct?
- Does he or she understand your needs?
- Does he or she ask about your expectations?
- Does he or she address your needs specifically and offer not only a recommended course of treatment, but also options that might be appropriate?
- Does he or she answer all of your questions directly, in a way that you fully understand?

- Has he or she, and/or the practice staff given you all the information you feel is important to make a decision?
- Has he or she addressed your budgetary concerns?

Another thing to review with a provider is his or her pre- and post-treatment photographs of similar cases. You should feel comfortable asking questions about the results in those photographs and how they were achieved.

In addition to credentials, experience, and outcomes, your personal experience is a very important factor in choosing a breast surgery provider. You should feel welcomed, comfortable, and secure in your provider's office. You should also be confident that you are safe and will be compassionately cared for.

12. What should I expect in a consultation?

Depending on the breast surgery you are considering or that has been prescribed, your initial visit or consultation may be somewhat different.

Plastic Surgery of the Breast

If you are electing to have plastic surgery of the breast to enhance the shape or appearance of your breasts, to improve your quality of life, or to treat disease, your initial visit with your plastic surgeon will be a consultation. You will meet with your plastic surgeon, and in many cases with a patient counselor or nurse who will guide you through the consultation process and subsequent **perioperative** course. However, you should never undergo any procedure without first meeting and consulting with the surgeon who will be treating you.

Perioperative

around the time of the surgery.

Most consultations begin by discussing your medical history, and your short- and long-term goals for plastic surgery of the breast. You will be asked specifically about what you wish to accomplish, and you will be informed about the treatments that can accomplish your goals. If you are not given photographic results of your recommended procedure(s) to review, you should ask to see pictures of the actual results the surgeon you are consulting with has achieved.

During your consultation, you will be examined so that your surgeon can evaluate your anatomy and physical condition, and determine how to best achieve your goals. Photographs of you will likely be taken for reference. The process of your procedure will also be discussed in detail.

During your consultation or in a subsequent visit, orders will be given for lab tests and medications. Specifics regarding anesthesia, location of procedures, itemized costs, patient obligations, and the recovery process will also be discussed. In addition, **sequelae**, which are the aftereffects or secondary results of your procedure, will be discussed. These include things you should expect as a result of the procedure, such as bruising and scars.

Sequelae

the aftereffects or secondary results of a surgical procedure.

Your physician should also directly define possible known risks, including unpredictable or unfavorable outcomes, and possible complications of the procedure you are considering. Despite a physician's personal safety record with any given procedure, known risks and complications must be fully disclosed. You will then be asked to sign informed consent documents.

All of the components of a plastic surgery consultation will occur during one or more visits, depending on your case and the physician's customary practices. A nurse or patient coordinator may guide you through the process. But decisions about procedures to be performed will be determined by you and the plastic surgeon.

Surgery to Diagnose or Treat Disease

You may find that your consultation experience with a general surgeon or plastic surgeon to diagnose or treat breast disease is very similar to that of a consultation for elective plastic surgery of the breast. In many cases, a nurse or patient advocate will guide you through the process. In all cases, your current and baseline test results should be available prior to or at the initial visit. Much like a plastic surgery consultation, your medical history will be discussed and condition examined.

Your surgeon may require additional testing prior to surgery, or the surgery may be diagnostic itself, for example, a needle biopsy. After the results are analyzed, your surgeon can then prescribe a course of treatment. This should include some insight as to the physical appearance and condition of your breast(s) following treatment, and the state of your health and general prognosis.

Unlike most plastic surgery consultations, taking photographs or reviewing photographs for reference is not regularly practiced. But don't overlook asking to see your surgeon's results, particularly if your breast surgery will be disfiguring. Surgeons with good aesthetic outcomes after **ablative breast surgery** (surgery to remove all or part of your breast; see Question 44) will likely be very pleased to share their results with you.

Ablative breast surgery

type of surgery to remove all or part of the breast.

When a course of treatment is prescribed, your focus will likely be on the prognosis of your health. But don't overlook asking specifically about what treatment for breast disease will do to the physical appearance of your breast, and about your options. For example, many women may be candidates for immediate **reconstruction** (reconstruction of the breast performed at the time of mastectomy) and by law have the right to insurance coverage for reconstruction (fully detailed in Question 49). Skin-sparing mastectomy and lumpectomy are also possible options (see Questions 42–47). Just as all physicians do not make it a practice to share photographs with you when treating breast disease, neither will all physicians discuss your options or your rights to reconstruction. You need to be your own best advocate and ask all the questions you want and need to have answered.

Reconstruction

a type of surgery to restore the breast at the time of or following mastectomy.

13. What are realistic goals?

Realistic goals mean that you fully understand what breast surgery can and cannot achieve for you. Before you make the decision or actually undergo breast surgery, ask yourself the following questions:

- Why do I want to have breast surgery?
- What do I specifically hope to accomplish through breast surgery?
- Do others see what I see and hope to improve through breast surgery?
- What is the risk to my health and my life by the treatment necessary to achieve what I want to accomplish, and am I willing to accept this risk?
- What expectations do I have for the physical outcome of breast surgery?

Where to Begin

- What are my expectations concerning my daily life?
- What are the expectations concerning my life, overall?
- Is my decision mine alone?
- Do those who support me in my daily life also support my desire for breast surgery?

Once you can answer these questions confidently, you and your surgeon together can determine if your goals are realistic. Realistic goals are defined as those that are both safe and attainable. In addition, realistic goals for aesthetic plastic surgery of the breast are:

- Not extreme
- Not the goals of anyone other than the patient
- Not life changing
- The goals of emotionally healthy individuals who want to improve their appearance for themselves

Beyond realistic goals, you must also consider realistic expectations for breast surgery. Realistic expectations include a complete understanding of the breast surgery process and accepting that process as necessary to achieve your realistic goals. The process of breast surgery, like any medical treatment or surgery, carries:

- Pretreatment and/or preoperative patient obligations
- Discomfort, anxiety, and pain
- Time commitment, downtime, and recovery
- Posttreatment and/or postoperative patient obligations
- Potential for unfulfilled goals and possible undesirable results
- Potential for physical risk
- Financial obligation, even with procedures that are not purely elective

Also, you need to understand that the difference between aesthetic plastic surgery of the breast and other medical treatments is that you are undergoing treatment by choice. Aesthetic surgery of the breast is not performed to promote better health. It includes a personal, emotional, and physical investment. You cannot expect to be fully satisfied by aesthetic surgery of the breast—even if the actual physical outcome was what you expected—unless you are prepared fully for the process that outcome will require.

I've been "overdeveloped" since the day I hit puberty. When I decided that the discomfort, restrictions to my life, and all the stares and glares were more than I could take, hearing someone ask me about my goals for breast reduction seemed ridiculous. I just want them smaller.

But realistic goals involve more than the outcome of breast surgery. Realistic goals involve accepting the process, the recovery, and the permanent change to your body. Once you understand what realistic goals are, and you know your goals are realistic, it makes the decision you face one of true confidence.

—Lauren, age 28, single

14. How do I communicate my expectations?

There is no better way in life to communicate anything than to do so directly. Ask questions when you need more information or do not understand something. Your consultation is the most important time to communicate your goals and expectations, that is, what you want to achieve and how you expect it will be accomplished.

Before your consultation or initial visit with your breast surgeon, it is a good idea to write down any questions you have. Your list should include questions about the procedure you are considering as well as questions about a provider's credentials and experience. In this way, you are less likely to overlook anything. Take this list with you to every consultation. Jot down information that you may wish to review with subsequent providers and compare the answers. You can also call a practice after your consultation if new questions arise.

Your expectations are not limited to the outcome of breast surgery, but also include the process. Tell the physician what you are willing to undergo in order to achieve your goals. Although you may be told your expectations are unrealistic, this doesn't mean you cannot continue to pursue your goals for breast surgery. It does mean that you must re-evaluate what you are willing to experience and accept less. You need to know what surgery and recovery entail, including the amount of time you need to recuperate. Make certain you are fully informed about possible complications as well.

15. Why are photographs necessary?

Photographs are necessary for physician reference in every case of plastic surgery of the breast. When performing plastic surgery of the breast, your surgeon needs to have a baseline visual anatomy of the areas to be treated. The photos are part of your medical record. These photos are important to you, too. To compare oneself before and after treatment in photographs taken in the same light, at the same angle, and same distance is truly an amazing experience.

But before any photograph of you is taken, even for your private patient record, you will likely be required to sign a release that specifically defines how and when a physician may use the photographs taken of you. When signing this release, recall how important it was for you to see the actual outcomes of other cases your physician performed. Realize that on the release form, you also may be asked to allow your photographs to be used for in-office patient education or other forms of patient education or research.

In addition to photographs taken in the physician's office, it is common for a patient to come into a consultation with photographs that illustrate what she wants to achieve. While bringing in a photograph of the size breasts you wish to have or of your breasts prior to ablative surgery may be helpful to visually express your goals, there is a caution. Your physician may not be able to meet the ideal of the photograph you present.

Very close to this issue is the debate about computer imaging and plastic surgery. Many professional societies have made strong statements against the use of computer imaging in a consultation. The reason is simple: given the nature of human anatomy and the physiology of healing, no result is fully predictable. While defining and planning breast size after surgery is one of the most easily controlled and achieved outcomes of any form of plastic surgery, don't believe for a minute that any physician can guarantee what your outcome will be.

I brought photographs of myself prior to having my kids to my consultation, so the doctor would believe I lost that much breast size. I never knew there would be pictures taken of me and my breasts during the consultation. But after surgery, when my doctor brought out my "before" pictures and then compared them to my "after" pictures, I was amazed and happy to be able to really see the difference breast surgery made for me.

—Kristin

16. What is informed consent?

Informed consent is a legal term, one that began in the 1950s to protect and educate people who volunteered to be the subjects of medical research. These documents were designed to explain:

Informed consent
the process a patient is taken through that defines a procedure prescribed to treat a condition, the risks and potential outcomes of the procedure, and a patient's potential alternatives.

- The nature of the research
- The specific anticipated outcomes
- The known risks
- That there was potential for unknown outcomes as risk factors
- That the research subject or patient, fully and voluntarily accepted all of the above

Today "informed consent" doesn't have a much different meaning than it had at its onset, but it is applied to many more situations than medical research. Informed consent is used with just about every form of medical treatment, except those cases that are life-threatening emergencies.

Informed consent for breast surgery of any kind, and particularly for elective breast surgery, is designed to make certain that you fully understand what to expect and that your physician is confident in your understanding. While many patients believe that informed consent is designed to protect the physician from being sued for negligence, no legal document can protect a physician from clear negligence. Make certain you understand all that a procedure or treatment entails as well as the possible risks and complications defined in an informed consent document, before signing the document.

PART THREE

Breast Surgery and Safety

Where is breast surgery performed?

What is accreditation and why is it important?

What are the risks of breast surgery?

More . . .

17. Where is breast surgery performed?

Breast surgery can be performed in any number of places.

Many diagnostic surgical procedures can be performed in an outpatient setting, as can lumpectomy, breast augmentation, breast lift, and some breast reductions. Significant breast reductions and any form of breast reconstruction should be performed in a hospital or ambulatory surgical facility that has appropriate accommodations where you can spend the night. The Breast Cancer Patient Protection Act of 2004 requires insurance companies to cover a minimum 48-hour hospital stay for patients undergoing a mastectomy.

Whether your procedure will be in an outpatient setting, ambulatory surgical facility, or hospital, make certain the facility where breast surgery is performed is fully **accredited** by a nationally recognized organization and/or is state licensed. This is essential to your safety.

Accreditation
a hospital, outpatient setting, or ambulatory surgical facility that has passed national and/or state regulated requirements for architecture, medical equipment, procedural protocols, and then inspection; must also adhere to all local, state, and national regulations including sanitation, fire safety, and building codes.

> In 2003, the American Society of Plastic Surgeons reported that 56% of all aesthetic procedures were performed in office-based surgical facilities, 28% were done in a hospital setting, and 16% in freestanding surgical facilities. This included breast surgery and other plastic surgery procedures.

18. What is accreditation and why is it important?

A physician must pass written and oral examinations to be board certified. Likewise, a facility must adhere to very specific requirements for architecture, medical equipment, procedural protocols, and then inspection to be granted accreditation. The following are accepted accrediting organizations for surgical facilities in the United States.

- The American Association for Accreditation of Ambulatory Surgery Facilities (AAAASF; *www.aaaasf.org*)
- The Accreditation Association for Ambulatory Health Care (AAAHC; *www.aaahc.org*)
- The Joint Commission on Accreditation of Healthcare Organizations (JCAHO; *www.jcaho.org*)
- Certification to participate in Medicare under title XVIII
- A state license to operate a medical facility, where required by state law

The Web sites of each of these organizations will give you specific requirements for accreditation and allow you to confirm the accreditation of a facility your physician recommends. In general, standards for accreditation include the following:

- Surgery is performed only by board-certified or board-eligible physicians of the American Board of Medical Specialties (ABMS) who hold privileges to perform the same procedures at a local, accredited hospital.
- Anesthesia is administered by only a board-certified or board-eligible anesthesiologist (physician) or certified registered nurse anesthetist (CRNA).
- Requirements for staff certification, namely surgical technicians, registered nurses, and licensed practical nurses, including training in advanced cardiac life support.
- The use of advanced monitoring during surgery and immediate recovery.

Furthermore, accreditation requires that a facility adhere to all local, state, and national regulations including sanitation, fire safety, and building codes. It also requires that the facility meet federal laws and Occupational Safety and Health Association (OSHA) regulations, including those for blood-borne pathogens and hazardous waste standards.

In addition to national, voluntary accreditation by the AAAASF, the AAAHC, and the JCAHO, some states require specific certification of facilities participating in Medicare billing. Also, accreditation is not always a substitute for state licensing of a surgical facility. Some states require licensing and others do not.

> In an effort to uphold the highest standards of safety for plastic surgery patients, since 2002 the American Society of Plastic Surgeons (ASPS) and the American Society for Aesthetic Plastic Surgery (ASAPS) mandated that all of their members operate in a hospital, state-licensed, or accredited facility.

19. What are the risks of breast surgery?

Infection
invasion of the body with organisms that have the potential to cause disease.

Pulmonary embolism
blockage of a lung artery; can be fatal.

Hematoma
a pooling of blood or fluid beneath the skin.

Breast surgery carries the same risks as any surgical procedure including: bleeding, **infection**, **pulmonary embolism**, anesthesia complications, and unexpected complications related to individual procedures. Understand that these risks are no greater for elective breast surgery patients than for patients undergoing any elective surgery.

Bleeding

Bleeding externally or under the skin (**hematoma**) can occur with any surgical procedure and can cause major problems. High blood pressure and medications (such as aspirin, ibuprofen, and some herbal supplements) can cause abnormal bleeding. If you have accidentally taken a medication that causes bleeding in the few weeks before surgery, be sure to tell your surgeon. You must tell your surgeon about all your medications and bleeding history. Your surgeon may ask for certain lab work to check your clotting ability. Some people have genetic bleeding disorders without a previous diagnosis.

Infection

Infection is possible with every surgery, even though strict sterile procedure is followed. You may, unknowingly, have an infection in your body or reduced ability to fight the small numbers of microorganisms in the air. Not all infection is the result of surgery, however. In fact, infection can occur long after surgery, during the healing process. Closely following your surgeon's instructions will not only help to avoid the risk of infection, but it will allow him or her to diagnose it early, when it is more easily controlled.

Embolism

Blood clots that can develop in the legs during or after surgery are among the most serious complications that can occur with surgery of any kind. These clots can lead to pulmonary embolism (blockage of a lung artery) and can be fatal. Careful patient selection through an evaluation of current health, use of medications and supplements, smoking habits, personal, and family health histories can help to identify those patients who are at greater risk.

Specific measures may be recommended to minimize the risk of blood clots, or you or your surgeon may decide the risks of surgery are too great and choose not to proceed with surgery. You can help to ensure your own safety by fully disclosing health history and following all instructions you are given.

Depending on the duration of the procedure, mechanical compression devices and/or antithrombotic medication may be used to help prevent emboli.

Anesthesia

Reactions to anesthesia can range from mild discomfort or irritation at a local anesthetic site, to nausea for sedation or with general anesthesia, to heart arrhythmia, and even death. Contemporary anesthesia equipment, however, has made surgery with sedation and general anesthesia much safer than in the past.

If your surgery is performed in an accredited freestanding facility, this equipment will have regular inspections to ensure that it is working properly. Furthermore, all accredited facilities have a protocol for immediate transfer to the nearest hospital if there is any serious problem.

Breast surgery carries some additional risks. In general these risks include a temporary or permanent loss of sensation in the breast, asymmetry, and risks related to procedural outcomes. The use of breast implants has the added risk of a condition of constricting excess scar tissue called capsular contracture. (Questions 36 and 37 discuss capsular contracture; all specific procedural risks are addressed in the definitions of breast surgery procedures within each section of this book.)

Scars are not a risk of breast surgery, but they are to be expected. However, how you heal and the formation of irregular scars is a risk that can be carefully controlled in many instances (see Questions 21, 22, and 96). A breast that does not fully appear or feel natural is also not a risk, but one of the trade-offs you must consider when electing some breast surgery procedures.

Statistics on **mortality** (death) demonstrate that surgery in an accredited, freestanding facility is as safe as a hospital. Based on a study conducted in 1997 by an independent group of physicians affiliated with the AAAASF and reported in the medical journal *Plastic and Reconstructive Surgery*:

- The rate of serious complications of plastic surgery procedures performed in accredited surgical facilities was less than one half of one percent (0.5%).
- The mortality rate was 1 in 57,000 cases.
- Infection was reported in 0.74% of cases.
- Patients required transfer to a hospital in 0.12% of cases.

20. Why will I need a physical, blood work, or pre-surgical testing?

Most breast surgery procedures are performed using intravenous or general anesthesia; in any non-emergency case, this requires that you undergo pre-surgical diagnostic testing. These tests are performed to detect possible health or bleeding problems, and even in the case of aesthetic breast surgery may be covered by your insurance.

Mortality
death.

Breast Surgery and Safety

Diagnostic testing may include:

- Blood count (**CBC**), blood chemistry, blood clotting tets, and possible screening for infectious diseases (such as hepatitis and HIV)
- A pregnancy test
- A chest x-ray and **electrocardiogram (ECG)** after a certain age, or if there is any pre-existing heart or lung disease
- A **mammogram** for most women above age 30–35 who are undergoing breast surgery and for any woman who is having breast surgery to diagnose or treat disease. (For women having breast implants for augmentation, a baseline mammogram is an important point of reference for future comparisons.)

In addition, patients with known medical problems or those beyond a certain age may require a report from an internist or general practitioner giving medical clearance for surgery.

If you are considering aesthetic breast surgery, don't look upon diagnostic testing as a nuisance or unnecessary expense. Medical testing gives your plastic surgeon the assurance that he or she will not likely cause harm by proceeding with surgery. In addition, the lab work may identify otherwise unknown, underlying medical problems that are readily treatable when caught early (such as high cholesterol).

21. What can I do to reduce my chance of health complications?

Choosing a qualified provider and an accredited surgical facility reduce your chance of complications. But you also have obligations as a patient. Your obligations as a patient will be carefully defined by your physician and include, but are not limited to:

- Correctly and fully disclosing your health history and that of your immediate family.
- Correctly and fully disclosing aspects of your lifestyle such as smoking and alcohol consumption, the use of prescriptive and other drugs, and the use of vitamins and herbal supplements.
- Listening carefully as instructions and the signs of complications are defined to you.
- Following instructions for pre-operative restrictions and purchases, diagnostic tests, etc.
- Reading, understanding, and following instructions for wound care, restrictions, medications, etc.
- Understanding all information regarding complications before your procedure so that you know what to look for and when to call your surgeon afterward.
- Recognizing and reporting any serious problems to your physician as soon as possible.
- Attending all pre-operative and post-operative appointments as scheduled.

Good Candidates

A good candidate for elective breast surgery is one who is motivated by his or her own desire, who has realistic expectations, and is in good health. The exception of a good candidate for prescribed breast surgery is that while breast health may be your goal and not your current condition, that maintaining overall health is indeed your goal as well.

What makes you a good *patient* is accepting responsibility for your health and safety. You must follow your physician's instructions precisely and inform your physician immediately if you develop any health problems either before or after your surgery.

It seems overwhelming – all the do's and don'ts you are given before and after surgery. But truly, to follow this was little commitment on my part to help my chances of avoiding risk and to having a good result.

—Lauren

22. Why am I told not to smoke or to avoid certain vitamins and medications?

Part of the education process before any surgery is to learn about those things that may harm you during surgery and/or the recovery phase. The physician, plastic surgeon, or his or her staff will provide you with detailed oral and written instructions about things you can do during your preparation weeks before surgery and during recovery that will help you be in the best possible health throughout the breast surgery process. Following these instructions precisely is important to preserving your health and achieving good outcomes.

Smoking

Human cells need oxygen to survive and reproduce, both of which are necessary factors in wound healing. Smoking reduces the amount of usable oxygen in the blood and constricts the vessels so that less blood is brought to the cells. With surgery, the number of vessels delivering blood to the wound is already reduced. Therefore, with smoking and surgery together, some cells are greatly deprived of oxygen and they die. The results are tissue that does not heal, infection, and large, unsightly scars. Furthermore, smoking diminishes lung capacity, so if you are to have sedation or general anesthesia, you may end up with severe respiratory problems including pneumonia.

Therefore, you will need to quit smoking several weeks prior to any elective surgical procedure and not smoke for several weeks afterward. If you are unable to quit smoking on your own, it is important to either get help or cancel surgery. If surgery is prescribed for you, quit smoking to protect your health. Your life may depend on it! By not disclosing to your surgeon that you are an active smoker, your risk of serious complications to your overall health and poor outcomes of surgery are significantly increased.

Medications, Vitamins, and Herbs

Your surgeon most likely will give you a list of medications to avoid before surgery. If some of them are prescriptions, your prescribing physician will need to give permission for you to stop taking these medications. He or she may also need to give you medical clearance before surgery.

In addition, some vitamins and herbal supplements can interfere with the ability of blood to clot properly, and can influence bruising and swelling. Be candid about any substances you take, and follow all instructions to discontinue these substances before and after surgery.

23. Can I choose where my procedure will be performed?

Generally, your surgeon will have a preference about where your surgery will be performed. If you are given a choice and safety is not an issue, then be sure you know the relative costs no matter if your procedure is elective or prescribed. Comparing prices in different facilities may save you money, but some insurers have requirements for coverage that define specifically where your procedure can be performed.

Recovery Choices

Today, few procedures require an overnight hospital stay. By law, however, mastectomy patients are permitted a two-night hospital stay (see Question 17). In most cases, you can recover comfortably at home with assistance from a friend, family member, or hired professional, or at an outpatient recovery facility.

Anesthesia

loss of physical sensation because of a pharmacologic depression of nerve function or neurologic dysfunction; broad term for anesthesiology as a clinical specialty.

Anesthesiologist

a physician specializing solely in anesthesiology and related areas, who is board-certified and legally qualified to administer anesthetics and related techniques.

Certified registered nurse anesthetist (CRNA)

a registered professional nurse with additional education and certification in the administration of anesthetics.

If you will not be staying in the hospital and you do not feel comfortable recovering at home, your surgeon may recommend a post-operative care facility that he or she believes is safe and expedient. Here you can recover in a setting that may be comfortable and private with some nursing care. It is always a good idea to visit the facility ahead of time and question the services, amenities, and costs. Then make your decision, based, of course, on your surgeon's recommendation.

24. What types of anesthesia will be used?

The types of **anesthesia** used in breast surgery depend upon the depth and extent of surgery and on your health. Your surgeon will give a recommendation and for some procedures there may be options available to you. You should also know the credentials of the person providing the anesthesia. With intravenous or general sedation, that person should be an **anesthesiologist** (medical doctor) or a **certified registered nurse anesthetist (CRNA)**.

The types of anesthesia used in breast surgery include:

- Oral
- Topical (cream and gel)
- Injectable (local or regional)
- **Intravenous (IV)** sedation (used with injectable anesthetics)
- General (with or without a tube in your trachea)

Intravenous (IV)
within a vein or
veins.

The anesthesia used will be based on your procedure and the recommendations of your surgeon and the anesthesiologist or nurse anesthetist. Your anesthesia options should be discussed with your plastic surgeon prior to surgery.

25. Can I choose what type of anesthesia will be used?

Your surgeon may give you some choices for anesthesia depending upon the procedure to be performed. For example, some procedures may be performed with general anesthesia or with local anesthesia and IV sedation (such as breast augmentation or breast lift), and you may have a choice of anesthesia in these cases. However, if your surgeon has a strong preference for one or the other, the anesthesia with which he or she is most comfortable should generally be used. Mastectomy and breast reduction are most commonly performed using general anesthesia, and there are very good reasons for doing so. You will be most comfortable during and after surgery when you are able to sleep soundly through the procedure.

Other procedures are commonly performed with local anesthesia alone, such as a needle biopsy. But, if you are anxious about surgery, you can ask for an oral medication to help you relax. If you are afraid of needles and scheduling a minor local procedure, you can also ask for a numbing cream prior to any injections.

PART FOUR

Breast Implants

What are breast implants?

When are breast implants used?

What types of breast implants are commonly used?

More . . .

26. What are breast implants?

Breast implants are medical devices that are surgically implanted into a woman's body to:

* Enhance and enlarge breast size and shape in breast augmentation
* Create the substance of a breast mound for breast reconstruction following mastectomy or other surgery to treat breast cancer
* Restore a more normal appearance to a woman's body that is lacking a breast due to congenital anomaly or birth defect

Breast implants were introduced in the United States in the early 1960s, mainly for augmentation purposes. It was not until 1976 that breast implants became subject to U.S. Food and Drug Administration (FDA) regulation under the U.S. FDA's Center for Devices and Radiological Health.

All breast implants currently in use in the United States are reviewed by the U.S. FDA Center for Devices and Radiological Health and are approved by the U.S. FDA. All approved breast implants have an outer shell of medical-grade, biocompatible solid silicone rubber.

* Implants approved strictly for enlargement or augmentation purposes are filled with sterile saline solution.
* Implants approved strictly for reconstructive purposes are saline or silicone filled.

In addition, silicone-filled implants are currently in clinical trails and pending U.S. FDA approval for augmentation. These implants were last reviewed for approval in April 2005.

Breast implants are surgically placed through incision patterns in a woman's body, either:

- Underneath existing breast tissue and on top of the chest muscles
- Beneath the chest muscles
- Beneath a muscle flap repositioned to the chest wall

There are several factors you must understand about all breast implants, and about all cases in which breast implants are placed into a woman's body.

First, know who is recommending and placing your breast implants. The only medical specialty with accredited training in breast surgery and the placement of breast implants is plastic surgery, and physicians who are certified by the American Board of Plastic Surgery. No other medical specialty has core training in breast surgery specific to the placement of breast implants.

Next, know that despite the fact that only board-certified plastic surgeons have the appropriate training to surgically place implants into your body, in the United States any licensed physician can purchase these medical devices and surgically implant them with your consent. It seems odd, but unfortunately medical manufacturers cannot deny selling these devices to a licensed physician. It would be a restraint of trade. Therefore, you must take it upon yourself to know exactly the qualifications and training of the physician who you will consult with and who will perform surgery to place breast implants into your body. You have the right and the responsibility to make certain of the surgeon's qualifications and expertise (see Questions 7–11).

Equally vital to your health and safety as knowing who will surgically place your implants is knowing what type of implants are being placed. Specific questions to ask include:

- The name of the manufacturer
- The type, model, and serial number

There are only two manufacturers of breast implants that are approved for use by the U.S. FDA in the United States: Inamed® Corporation (who acquired McGahn Medical) and Mentor® Corporation. If the breast implants recommended for your surgery are not manufactured by either of these two companies, you must ask some very serious questions of your surgeon. Either the implants being used are part of an U.S. FDA-qualified clinical trial and so you will be a research subject or, more likely, the implants being used are an imported device and not subject to U.S. FDA regulation. Be cautious. Imported devices may be cheaper, but they have no proven track record for safety or outcomes in the United States. Therefore, you should not agree to the use of any implant that is not manufactured by Inamed® or Mentor®, or that is not part of a qualified U.S. FDA trial.

The American Society of Plastic Surgeons and the American Society for Aesthetic Plastic Surgery have made statements advising their members against the use of imported medical devices and substances. However, no public policy exists that prohibits or makes it unlawful to use imported medical devices with a patient's consent.

Both Inamed® Corporation and Mentor® Corporation have Web sites specific to breast implants and breast implant surgery. Visit *www.inamed.com* and *www. mentorcorp.com* for more information about their breast implants, breast augmentation, and breast reconstruction. In addition, the American Society of Plastic Surgeons (*www.plasticsurgery.org*) and the American Society for Aesthetic Plastic Surgery (*www.surgery.org*) have online information about all breast implants and their use in women.

27. When are breast implants used?

Whether for augmentation or reconstruction purposes, breast implants are only used when a woman chooses them. Even when they are prescribed to improve the proportion of a woman's figure, to reconstruct a breast, or to achieve symmetry between a breast that has been reconstructed and a natural breast, there is no reason a woman *must* undergo surgery to place breast implants.

Breast implants can have an immensely positive influence on a woman's self-esteem and self-image. But breast implants do not treat disease, nor are they essential to a woman's health or treatment outcomes. Therefore, the placement of breast implants in your body is entirely by choice, even when implants are part of a prescribed breast reconstruction. You may be supported and encouraged by those whom you love, by your plastic surgeon, and other physicians in your consideration of breast implants. But the bottom line is that choosing breast implants is a decision you must make for yourself, by yourself.

There are alternatives to breast implants. In the case of augmentation, a woman may choose to wear padded bras, she may choose to pad her bra with external **prosthetic enhancements**, or she may choose to simply accept her breasts as they are.

Prosthetic enhancements
artificial parts of the body that help the figure to appear more natural; are removable.

In some cases of breast reconstruction, specialized plastic surgery techniques that rebuild a woman's breast using her own muscle and/or fat and skin may be an alternative to the use of breast implants. A woman may choose to wear prosthetic bras or pad her bra with external prosthesis, or she may choose to accept her condition and live with the absence or deformity of her breast. But these alternatives are not right for everyone. Prosthetic solutions have their limitations in fashion choices and to a woman's self-image. The only true fulfillment you may feel is through seeing yourself as you feel your breasts and your body should be. If that is the case, the choice for breast implants must be your decision.

With rare exception, implants should **not** be placed into a woman's body if she is pregnant or nursing, if she has an active infection or critical illness present anywhere in the body, or if she has an existing malignant or pre-malignant breast cancer that is not being treated. An exception is infection surrounding an existing breast implant, in which case the course of treatment may include removing or occasionally replacing an implant. In addition, women with certain medical conditions that may impair healing may be advised not to consider breast implants. The U.S. FDA has only approved breast implants strictly for augmentation purposes (to cosmetically enhance size) for women age 18 or older. Augmentation candidates who have emotional or psychological conditions such as **body dysmorphic disorder (BDD)** will likely be referred for counseling prior to breast implant surgery.

Body dysmorphic disorder is a very serious psychological condition noted to be similar to obsessive-compulsive disorder. It is a preoccupation with an imagined physical defect or a vastly exaggerated concern about a minimal defect. Individuals with BDD are so troubled by the perceived defect that they obsess over it for more than one hour per day. BDD should only be diagnosed by a licensed and appropriately trained psychologist or psychiatrist; it should not be a label used by opponents of plastic surgery or breast implants. In fact, in a study conducted by the American Society for Aesthetic Plastic Surgery in 2003, their members report less than 2% of patients who consult with them exhibit symptoms of BDD. ASAPS members and plastic surgeons in the study also responded that 84% refused to perform surgery on patients who displayed symptoms of BDD and the majority referred these patients for counseling.

There have been external medical devices, exercises, herbal supplements, and creams touted to increase breast size. In fact, these substances may be harmful to a woman's health as they are not reviewed or approved by the FDA. However, nothing has the proven satisfaction and outcomes of breast implants in breast augmentation. The use of breast implants in augmentation

Body dysmorphic disorder (BDD)
a psychosomatic (an influence of the mind about the body) characterized by a preoccupation with some imagined defect in appearance in a normal-appearing person.

Breast Implants

surgeries, as reported by the American Society of Plastic Surgeons in 2003, was just over 250,000 cases (not implants). This is a greater than 600% increase in the use of breast implants for augmentation purposes since 1992.

28. What types of breast implants are commonly used?

All breast implants currently in use in the United States, and reviewed by the U.S. Food and Drug Administration (FDA) Center for Devices and Radiological Health and approved by the U.S. FDA, have an outer shell made of medical-grade, biocompatible, solid silicone rubber. These implants are either filled with a sterile saline solution, or those approved strictly for reconstructive purposes may be silicone filled or a combination of silicone-filled with a saline core for tissue expansion. In addition, silicone filled implants are currently in clinical trials and are pending U.S. FDA approval for use in augmentation.

Implants vary not only in their composition, but also by size, shape, and other factors. Breast implants are also characterized by:

- The size of the implant, typically measured by the volume of the substance filling the implant
- The projection or profile of the implant, in variations from low to high
- The dimensions of the implant measured by base diameter and projection
- The shell of the implant: smooth or textured, and always of silicone rubber

Silicone-filled implants are always pre-filled. Saline-filled implants may be pre-filled, or filled at the time of placement into a woman's body. Silicone and saline implants are additionally characterized by the shape of the implants. Some are round and others are contoured with varying degrees in profile.

The differences among implants result in more than just an enhancement of breast size. The type of implant used can:

- Enhance overall breast size (width) and projection
- Enhance the projection of a well-rounded, yet flat breast
- Enhance the overall size and width of a small breast with good projection
- Create cleavage
- Reconstruct a proportionate breast to a woman's body, with a very natural shape and slope

Women's bodies vary greatly, as do their goals for how breast implants will improve one's body image. Therefore, it is essential that prior to any breast implant being recommended in your case, your plastic surgeon or his or her nurse examine you, take photographs, and possibly take measurements of your current breast profile. In addition, you should be clear on your goals, and define exactly how you wish to see yourself following the placement of breast implants.

Both Inamed® and Mentor® keep up-to-date Web sites with all currently available breast implant models listed. For more information, visit *www.inamed.com* and *www.mentorcorp.com*.

If you are considering breast implants and have concerns about latex allergies, you can be confident that the implant shells in use today are latex-free. Inamed® offers information specific to latex concerns on their consumer Web site, *www.inamed.com.*

In 1996, the Trilucent™ implant, filled with purified soybean oil was introduced. In the United States about 200 women received this implant in a U.S. FDA-approved, controlled research study. The study was ended in 1997, due to complications associated with the implant. In June 2000, the Medical Devices Agency (MDA) in the United Kingdom issued a warning entitled *Trilucent™ Breast Implants: Recommendation to Remove*, advising women with Trilucent™ Breast Implants worldwide to have them removed even if they are not experiencing complications. Although not manufactured or marketed by Inamed Corp. or McGahn®, Inamed® does have information specific to the Trilucent implant on their Web site, *www.inamed.com.*

Silicone- and saline-filled implants are not the only implants you may hear or read about. Manufacturers and plastic surgeons all over the world are testing all sorts of new breast implant fillers. In early 2004, the same researchers who had introduced and tested Trilucent™ breast implants in 1996 had patented a breast implant filled with polyethelene glycol and saline, and applied to the U.S. FDA to begin using it in clinical trials. In addition, hyaluronic acid-filled implants are in research and development. It is likely that other combinations of substances are under study throughout the world, or currently are being developed.

29. When is a pre-filled implant used versus one that is not pre-filled?

In most cases, the decision to use an implant that is filled at the time of placement into a woman's body is based on:

- Surgical method and incision pattern used to place the implant
- A need to adjust implant size to achieve a more uniform result in disproportionate breasts
- Your plastic surgeon's preference

Remember that only saline-filled implants can be filled at the time of surgery to place them. But just as pre-filled implants have a defined size, implants filled at the time of surgery do have a defined range of saline based on the implant size. Implants that are underfilled may result in wrinkling or drooping, and implants that are overfilled may have a distinctly unnatural fullness, be easily **palpable** (felt by touching with hands) under the breast tissue, and feel much firmer than natural breast tissue. Therefore, it is imperative that you ask your surgeon specifically what type of breast implants he or she will use in your case, about his or her experience with those implants, and the reasons for recommending them to you.

Palpable

capable of being felt in an examination by the hands.

Do not confuse an implant filled at time of placement with one that is initially used as a tissue expander. In cases where ample tissue does not exist at the breast mound to cover a breast implant (most commonly in the case of breast reconstruction), a saline-filled breast implant may first serve as a tissue expander. The process of tissue expansion requires the implant to be slowly filled with sterile saline over many weeks and

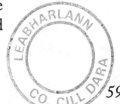

Breast Implants

multiple visits to your plastic surgeon's office. Many of these implants have self-sealing valves and, therefore, are left in place once the desired size is reached, or they may be replaced with another type of implant after the tissue expansion process is completed.

30. What is the difference between silicone- and saline-filled implants?

The most common distinction and greatest debate among breast implants today is whether they are filled with saline or with silicone. Each type of implant filler has unique characteristics that offer advantages and considerations for use. Before you consider the differences between silicone- and saline-filled implants, you need to understand exactly the parameters for use of these implants.

Silicone-filled implants, as of the writing of this book, are only used in the United States in breast reconstruction cases, in specific research studies, or to replace existing silicone implants. In October 2003, a U.S. FDA advisory panel recommended reinstatement of silicone breast implants based on a petition filed by Inamed® Corp. for a new generation of cohesive silicone-filled breast implants, as an option to any women seeking breast augmentation. As of the publication of this book, the U.S. FDA has chosen to wait for the results from more long-term clinical studies before accepting the petition and giving approval with subsequent review scheduled for April 2005. Mentor® Corporation has also filed for review and approval specific to breast augmentation of their version of the cohesive silicone-filled breast implant.

Character and Considerations

Silicone breast implants, both the earlier and newer generations, have a more natural appearance and feel than do saline breast implants. For this reason, they are highly preferred by both surgeons and women, particularly in breast reconstruction where little of a woman's own soft tissue is present to cover and cushion the breast implant. In addition, the newest generation of silicone-filled implants come in a greater variety of contours (shapes) and therefore are more likely to result in more natural physical outcome. The earlier generation of silicone-filled implants had a somewhat higher rate of a complication called **capsular contracture**; however, this has not proven to be the case with currently available silicone implants. However, capsular contracture can be worsened in many women by the lack of soft tissue to cover the implant. This complication results in varying degrees of breast hardness and deformity, and is fully discussed in Questions #36 and #37.

Saline implants do have a feel that is firmer and more palpable (more easily felt). But saline implants do not have as broad a range in shape and design. It is, however, a myth that an appropriately filled saline breast implant can make a sloshing noise as a woman moves her body. All saline implants will wrinkle, even if overfilled. Wrinkling may be visible, particularly where little or no breast tissue is available to provide implant coverage. These characteristics are generally not visible with clothing and rarely noticeable to other individuals. In addition, implants with a textured shell are more likely to wrinkle than implants with a smooth shell.

Capsular contracture
when excess scar tissue constricts over time; may occur with breast implants.

Breast Implants

If saline implants should leak or rupture, the sterile saline solution they are filled with is safely absorbed and expelled by the body. You will notice if your saline-filled implant is leaking or ruptured, as your breast will slowly or rapidly deflate. Removal and replacement of a saline implant is a relatively minor surgical procedure when treated early. While it is to your best advantage to have the ruptured or leaking saline-filled implant removed or replaced as soon as possible, there is no apparent threat to your health.

If silicone-filled implants rupture or leak, you may not notice it right away, and it is possible that the leaking silicone can cause pain or deformity. This was particularly the case for silicone breast implants prior to the newly introduced generation of cohesive silicone implants. The most effective non-surgical means to determine if a silicone implant is leaking is through **magnetic resonance imaging (MRI)**. If a silicone implant is determined to be leaking, it should be surgically removed as soon as possible. Free silicone from leaking or ruptured implants can potentially migrate outside the breast capsule and into the body, and as much of it as possible should be removed to avoid hard nodules called **granulomas**. The procedure can be very involved and results in a significant recovery time.

Your choice of implants is best determined by discussing your options with your surgeon. Considerations include your lifestyle, the amount of enhancement you desire, and your personal preferences. To fully understand what implants will be used in your case, always request to examine the implant package insert from your plastic surgeon prior to sur-

Magnetic resonance imaging (MRI)

a type of diagnostic radiologic technique using nuclear magnetic resonance technology to provide three-dimensional pictures from inside of a body to check for health and disease.

Granulomas

nodular inflammatory lesions, usually small or granular, firm, persistent, and containing compactly grouped cells.

gery. Following your surgery, your plastic surgeon should give you the implant manufacturer's device information. Keep this information in a safe place. It identifies the brand of implant you received, its size, the manufacturer's lot number, and its warranty. Should your implants ever need to be replaced, this information is very important.

According to data published by the U.S. Food and Drug Administration Center for Devices and Radiological Health, the following breast implants have greater palpability, that is, they are felt more easily: textured implants, larger implants, **sub-glandularly placed implants** (on top of the chest muscle, below the breast glands), and implants in patients with smaller amounts of breast tissue.

Sub-glandularly placed implants
type of implants placed on top of the chest muscle and below the breast glands.

31. Why were silicone-gel-filled breast implants recalled in the 1990s?

In the early 1990s silicone-gel-filled breast implants were voluntarily suspended from the market by breast implant manufacturers at the request of the U.S. FDA. At issue was the theory that these implants contributed to connective tissue or autoimmune diseases (such as rheumatoid arthritis, lupus, and chronic fatigue syndrome) in some women. The U.S. FDA action was specific to the use of silicone-gel-filled implants in breast augmentation only, and implant manufacturers voluntarily took their silicone-gel-filled implants off the market, pending safety review. However, some silicone-gel-filled implants have remained an available option for breast reconstruction patients with specific procedural protocols, and for patients in formal research studies.

After multiple lawsuits and credible independent research by the Institute of Medicine (IOM), the U.S. FDA published the *Breast Implants Information Update 2000*. This document cites the highly regarded IOM studies that dispelled possible links to illness and silicone breast implants in some women. The IOM independent scientific panel found that silicone breast implants do not increase the risk or signs and symptoms of autoimmune diseases in women as some legal claims stated. Specifically, the report stated, "It is unclear at this time whether the signs and symptoms experienced by these women are related to their implants."

The findings of several other independent studies are also reported in the U.S. FDA *Update*, including one of the most comprehensive, performed by researchers at Harvard Medical School in 1996. This study reported, "A small but statistically insignificant risk of all CTDs (connective tissue disorders) reported by women with breast implants...over a 10-year period, women with breast implants were 1.24 times more likely to report having a CTD or related disorder." The U.S. FDA summarized all of the studies they reviewed, stating, "When considered together, these studies indicate that the risk of developing a typical or defined CTD or related disorder due to having breast implants is low."

In 2003, a U.S. FDA advisory panel reviewed a petition from breast implant manufacturer Inamed® Corporation to market a newer generation of silicone breast implant, one filled with "cohesive" silicone. In October 2003, the panel voted and recommended that the U.S. FDA should approve, with conditions, their implant for use in breast reconstruction, breast augmentation, and revisional breast surgery procedures. In January 2004, the U.S. FDA did not, however, act upon the advisory panel's recommendation, pending further information from Inamed.® Mentor® Corporation has since submitted their version of the cohesive silicone breast implant for U.S. FDA review and approval.

The U.S. FDA established MedWatch to report "adverse events" thought to be associated with medical devices or drugs. With regard to silicone-gel-filled breast implants, if you experience a serious adverse effect that you and your physician believe is related to your breast implant, your surgeon should complete a MedWatch Form 3500, provide you with a copy, and submit the document to the U.S. FDA. Medwatch forms are available at *http://www.fda.gov/medwatch/index.html.*

32. How do the silicone implants used today differ from those used in the past?

Not all of the silicone implants used today differ from those used in the past. It is the newly developed "cohesive" silicone implants that differ greatly. Cohesive means that the silicone with which the implants are filled is binding unto itself and is therefore unlikely to migrate should the implants leak or rupture. Some journalists and physicians have named these "gummy" implants because they have characteristics similar to the gummy bear candies. When cut in half, the highly cohesive implants remain soft and pliable without anything leaking or dripping out. You must understand that this is not a fair characterization of all cohesive implants, as there has been no accepted standard set to define what is cohesive. The newer generation of silicone implants has a shell that is less likely to allow silicone to sweat or bleed through, and this also reduces the chance of capsular contracture.

Your best ability to judge whether you will feel comfortable with the silicone implant recommended in your case is to ask to see that implant, and if possible compare the silicone and saline implants.

33. How do I determine if silicone- or saline-filled, or any implants are right for me?

It is your right to have breast implants, just as it is your right to accept any form of medical treatment. Research and the media should not influence your decision. They merely provide you with information. Be cautious of where your research is gathered, and who may be influencing the information you obtain. Information does not come with instructions, so here are some guidelines for using all the information you obtain and for making a decision about breast implants that is right for you.

Use media as a source for questions, but not answers. Obtain your answers from a board-certified plastic surgeon and review the results of research published by unbiased patient advocate groups, such as the U.S. FDA, the National Institutes of Health (NIH), the Institute of Medicine (IOM), and recognized medical specialty societies such as the American Society of Plastic Surgeons (ASPS).

Visit the Web sites of breast implant manufacturers or ask your plastic surgeon for specific data on the breast implants you are considering, published by the manufacturer of that breast implant. All public information published or advertised by a pharmaceutical company or a medical device manufacturer is subject to U.S. FDA review. These companies can be fined or have their products pulled from the market if they release false or biased information. A new Web site, *www.breastimplant.org,* has specific information regarding the safety of breast implants and is endorsed by the American Society of Plastic Surgeons and the American College of Surgeons.

Now, take all of your research and all of your questions with you to your office visit, and have a discussion with a qualified, board-certified plastic surgeon with whom you feel comfortable and confident. Also, talk with your personal physician if you wish. Gynecologists see only female patients, including those with breast implants. It is useful to talk with other women who have breast implants. If you don't know someone who has breast implants, ask your surgeon or gynecologist for references to patients who do have implants, and talk to these women.

If you truly have the desire for breast augmentation or reconstruction using implants, make no decision until you go through the process of informed consent with your plastic surgeon. The process of informed consent is fully discussed in Question 16. It is your right to

Breast Implants

choose to have breast implants. Make certain your decision is purely your own.

For access to current information on breast implants visit:

www.fda.gov, U.S. FDA Center for Devices and Radiological Health, breast implants

www.nih.gov, and search on the homepage for breast implants

www.iom.edu, and search under Women's Health for breast implants

www.breastimplantsafety.org

www.plasticsurgery.org, and search for breast implants

www.inamed.com, and click on the link to breast augmentation or breast reconstruction

www.mentor.com, and click on the link to breast surgery

34. Can breast implants cause breast disease or negatively affect my health?

There is no proven link between any form of breast surgery, including surgery with implants, and breast disease. The National Institutes of Health (NIH) and National Cancer Institute (NCI), and the U.S. Food and Drug Administration (FDA) at the time of publication of this book had no statement linking breast implants or breast surgery to breast disease, nor did they report data linking women who have undergone breast surgery for implants to breast disease.

In 2000, the U.S. Institute of Medicine reported that breast cancer is no more common in women with implants than those without implants. In addition, in April 2001, researchers at the NCI issued a report stating that, "women with silicone breast implants were not at increased risk for most cancers." Their study specifically stated that no increased risk was found for sarcoma, Hodgkin's or non-Hodgkin's lymphoma, or multiple myeloma.

With regard to illnesses other than breast cancer, the U.S. FDA Center for Devices and Radiological Health reported in 2000 that most studies of the illnesses believed to be linked to breast implants, "have failed to show an association with breast implants." Further, the same report offers that there is no information that breast implants may be damaging to children born of mothers with implants (silicone gel or saline filled), who breast-fed or did not.

However, studies do suggest that breast implants in some cases can impede the ability of a woman to breastfeed. How often this occurs is not known. More importantly, research reported by the U.S. FDA in 1998 found that silicone levels in breast milk of women with silicone-gel-filled breast implants were the same when compared with breast milk from women without implants.

Capsular contracture is the only breast condition unquestionably linked to breast implants. Capsular contracture is not breast disease, however, but excess scar tissue that forms around the implant. The condition can occur with any type of implanted device in the body, and it can be minimized and corrected in nearly every case.

Having breast implants, in fact, can have advantages that reach beyond a woman's own confidence with her body image. Women who have had breast surgery of any kind are more likely to practice breast self-examination (BSE) and to be more in tune with the feel and form of their breast tissue. In a report by the Mayo Clinic, women with saline breast implants found it easier to do breast self-exam. The implants separated breast tissue from the body, making changes in breast tissue more apparent.

Therefore, you should not base your decision for breast implants on the unproven notion that having breast implants can impair your health.

35. Can having breast implants cause any form of disease or affect my overall health?

Published reports from the U.S. FDA Center for Devices and Radiological Health, the National Institutes of Health, and the independent Institute of Medicine have found that no forms of disease are caused by breast implants.

However, breast implants can interfere with two key means to diagnose breast cancer:

- Mammography
- Sentinel node biopsy

Mammography in women with breast implants must be performed at a certified mammography center with personnel having experience in taking and reading mammograms of women with breast implants. First, the compression necessary to take a mammogram film presents a risk of rupturing your implants. This is rare, and more likely occurs when the breast implant has a firm capsule of scar tissue surrounding it. It is important to tell the mammography center you have breast implants when scheduling your mammogram.

Additionally, breast implants can make screening a mammogram more difficult, because the implant can block the ability to see all areas of breast tissue. As a result, it is possible that areas with breast disease may be present, but are hidden from view. To avoid the potential of an incomplete or inaccurate screening, additional mammography views will likely be required.

Sentinel node biopsy is a surgical procedure performed to determine if breast cancer has spread to adjoining lymph nodes. In this procedure, a dye is injected around a tumor before it is completely removed. The dye is carried from the area of the tumor to the lymph nodes where the cancerous cells of the tumor may be likely to have spread. Currently available research suggests that the surgical placement of breast implants should not impair your ability to have an accurate sentinel node biopsy, with the possible exception of the transaxillary incision.

In addition, certain incision patterns to place breast implants, namely those around the **areola** (the dark tissue surrounding the nipple) and those in the **axilla** (the underarm area) may interfere with sentinel node biopsy and the diagnosis of cancerous cells in the lymph nodes. These incision patterns may cut or interrupt the lymphatic drainage channels and prevent the dye from spreading to lymph nodes where cancer may, in fact, have spread. There are alternatives, and you must discuss these with your surgeon prior to any procedure to diagnose or treat breast cancer, benign cysts, or tumors.

Sentinel node biopsy
surgical procedure performed to determine if breast cancer has spread to adjoining lymph nodes.

Areola
the dark tissue surrounding the nipple of the breast.

Axilla
the underarm area.

In addition, radiation therapy to treat breast cancer or other cancers localized near the breast may damage the tissue surrounding your breast implant, and cause an unnatural firmness and irregular shape to your breast.

With regard to your overall health, breast implants can result in complications that affect your life, and thus your overall health. The potential for these risks are a trade-off you must consider in your personal fulfillment to enhancing or restoring your breast through the placement of breast implants.

36. What are the possible risks of breast implants?

The possible risks related to the use of breast implants include the risks of surgery in general, the risks of breast surgery in general, and risks related to the type of implant and its physical placement at the breast site.

Risks related to surgery include the risks related to anesthesia. Risks following surgery include infection, hematoma (pooling of blood beneath the skin), and the formation of blood clots. These risks can occur with any form of surgery, not just surgery to place breast implants. Any sign of infection must be reported immediately to your plastic surgeon. If not treated effectively, infection may lead to wound-healing problems or a loss of healthy tissue, which is called **necrosis**. Poor wound healing and necrosis are more likely if you:

Necrosis

death of one or more cells, or of a portion of tissue or organ, that may result in permanent damage (such as scar tissue). The loss of skin or tissue due to a lack of blood supply or infection.

* Have been using steroid drugs
* Are undergoing chemotherapy
* Have undergone radiation to the breast tissue

- Are a smoker
- Have used excessive heat or cold on healing wounds

Risks related to any form of breast surgery include a change in the sensation of the breast or nipple, an impaired ability to breast-feed, and breast tenderness.

Risks related to breast implants specifically include:

- Wrinkling of implants
- Palpability (how it feels under the skin)
- Asymmetry between the breasts
- Capsular contracture
- Calcification
- Ruptured or leaking implants
- Implant displacement
- Implant extrusion

Breast implant wrinkling is possible with all breast implants, particularly with saline implants that have been underfilled. The condition is likely not visible under clothing. Surgical replacement may be recommended in severe and visible cases of wrinkling. Much like wrinkling, breast implant palpability is a condition likely only detectable to the woman with breast implants. Palpability is described as the condition where the implant can be easily felt under the beast tissue or chest muscle. Like wrinkling, only replacement and repositioning the breast implant pocket under the chest muscle can minimize this condition.

Capsular contracture results when the naturally formed capsule of tissue around the implant becomes irregularly firm or tightens. Where contracture is excessive, the capsule can squeeze the breast and result in a change to the breast shape and/or position, and in some cases may even cause discomfort. Capsular contracture is more likely with sub-glandular placement of breast implants (under the breast tissue and above the chest muscle), with silicone implants, and with larger implants where little breast tissue covers the implant. Capsular contracture sometimes may be the result of previous bleeding or a low-grade infection. Where a woman has had breast implants placed uniformly at each breast, the condition may not develop uniformly. In fact, it may develop on one breast and not the other.

Breast implants also have the potential risk to leak or rupture. This may happen suddenly as the result of trauma to the breast, or for no apparent reason at all.

Calcification is a condition where calcium deposits develop around the breast implant capsule, causing firmness and occasionally pain. This is not capsular contracture, as the deposits are localized and they do not affect the entire breast. In addition, where calcium deposits cannot be differentiated from those that are early signs of breast cancer, they must be removed and examined to ensure your health, and to prevent damage to the breast implant.

Displaced implants can only be corrected surgically. **Symmastia** is a condition where the capsule or pocket in which breast implants are placed is too close, or where the breast implants displace into one large pocket. The result is that the implants actually meet in the middle of the chest and appear to be one big breast. Correction of symmastia requires that the breast pocket be internally and permanently sutured smaller,

Calcification

a condition where calcium deposits develop around the breast implant capsule, causing firmness and occasionally pain.

Symmastia

a condition where the capsule or pocket in which breast implants are placed is too close, or where the breast implants displace into one large pocket, resulting in implants that meet in the middle of the chest and appear to be one big breast. Correction requires that the breast pocket be internally and permanently sutured smaller, and that implants be replaced and repositioned.

and that implants be replaced and repositioned. Symmastia must be addressed by a plastic surgeon qualified and experienced in treating this condition.

Extrusion is an extreme risk where a breast implant may actually break through to the skin surface and become exposed. This condition is very rare, and must be evaluated immediately, because it can result in permanent scarring and loss of healthy breast tissue and skin.

Changes in your breast shape and appearance as you age and that result from pregnancy or weigh fluctuations are not a risk of breast implants. This can happen to women who don't have breast implants. In fact, the insertion of breast implants may, in fact, allow your breasts to retain their shape better over time than a natural breast.

According to data published by the U.S. Food and Drug Administration (FDA) Center for Devices and Radiological Health, the following implants are reported to be more palpable (more easily felt): textured implants, larger implants, sub-glandularly placed implants (on top of the chest muscle, below the breast glands), and implants in patients with smaller amounts of breast tissue. The U.S. FDA also reported that there is no greater risk of capsular contracture with textured implant shells than smooth-shelled implants.

37. How is capsular contracture corrected?

Your plastic surgeon will likely diagnose your capsular contracture based on its grade in what is called the **Baker scale**:

- Grade I: The breast is normally soft and looks natural

Extrusion
where a breast implant actually breaks through to the skin surface and becomes exposed.

Baker scale
a standardized test to measure capsular contracture varying from Grade I (breast is normally soft and natural appearing) to Grade IV (breast is very firm, with clearly visible distortion in shape, and the patient may experience pain).

Breast Implants

- Grade II: The breast is somewhat firm but remains normal in appearance
- Grade III: The breast feels firmer than normal and has some changes in shape
- Grade IV: The breast is very firm, with clearly visible distortion in shape, and the patient may experience pain

Early, mild cases of capsular contracture can be reduced with breast massage and/or minimal surgical release. However, in Grade III and IV cases, contracture may be so severe that the scar tissue needs to be removed and the implant replaced. Even if the implant is replaced, capsular contracture can reoccur.

Closed capsulotomy

a controversial technique that is not recommended to treat capsular contracture; involves a very forceful squeezing of the breast capsule to release or tear it; can result in implant rupture and localized bleeding, and may void the breast implant manufacturer's warranty.

A **closed capsulotomy** is a technique that is not recommended to treat capsular contracture. This involves a very forceful squeezing of the breast capsule to release or tear it. This technique is highly controversial as it can result in implant rupture and localized bleeding. Be advised that having a closed capsulotomy may in fact void your breast implant manufacturer's warranty.

38. How are leaking or ruptured implants treated?

The only means to treat leaking or ruptured implants of any kind is through surgical removal, and replacement with another breast implant appropriately recommended for you.

Leaking silicone-filled implants may be detected by decreased breast size, hard knots in the breast, uneven appearance of the breasts, swelling, tenderness, numbness or burning, or the development of significant capsular contracture. However, the best currently available test to determine whether your silicone implants are leaking is magnetic resonance imaging (MRI). It is recommended that leaking or ruptured silicone implants of any kind be removed even if the silicone is contained.

Saline implants simply deflate when they are ruptured or leaking, and are therefore easy to recognize and simple to replace if treated early. Again, these implants may only be replaced surgically.

Any woman who chooses only to have a leaking or ruptured implant removed but not replaced faces the possibility of highly disfigured breasts. Once the breast implant that provided volume for your breasts is no longer present, you will likely have flat, droopy breasts. Literally, they will have the appearance of an outstretched and empty pocket. Problems of drooping breasts and dimpled or puckered breast skin can only be corrected through additional surgery, the outcomes of which may be highly variable.

Implant manufacturers' warranties may cover the cost of implant replacement in certain cases, and contribute to the cost of anesthesia fees and operating room facilities. Read your implant warranty carefully to understand exactly what it covers and how you can claim benefits.

According to the American Society of Plastic Surgeons and the American Society for Aesthetic Plastic Surgery publication, *Silicone Breast Implant Surgery: Information for Women,* breast implant manufacturers' statistics demonstrate a re-operation rate for breast implants of 20%–30% after five years for breast augmentation patients, and 30%–40% after five years for breast reconstruction patients.

39. Is there any other reason why my implants may need to be replaced?

Leaking or ruptured implants are not the only reason for implant replacement. Capsular contracture may require implant replacement as well as any other risks associated with breast implants.

More commonly though, women choose to have their breast implants replaced when:

- A woman desires a change in her breast size
- Newer types of breast implants that offer the advantages a woman desires become available
- The nature of a woman's body and breasts change somewhat, and she chooses to replace her implants to maintain the body image she desires
- Your plastic surgeon recommends having your implants replaced

The U.S. FDA defines that breast implants are not lifetime devices. Whether you choose to have your implants replaced, or for any reason your plastic surgeon recommends they be replaced, you must accept that it is likely in your lifetime that your implants will be replaced.

Even if you are experiencing no complications of any kind with your implants, it is wise to have your plastic surgeon evaluate the condition of your implants as he or she recommends. This can be done in a simple, in-office examination that takes only a few minutes.

Having breast implants is a lifetime decision, and it also offers a lifetime of personal reward. Take the time to ensure the health and condition of your breasts and your breast implants. The investment in your time is minimal compared to complications that can result.

In 2003, ASPS reported that 45,147 of the breast implants done for augmentation purposes only, were removed, of which 81% were replaced. The most common reasons for implant removal were (1) a change in breast size, and (2) implant rupture or leakage.

PART FIVE

Treating Breast Disease

How does breast surgery treat disease?

Is breast surgery used strictly to treat breast cancer?

What is a lumpectomy or breast conserving surgery?

More . . .

40. How does breast surgery treat disease?

In the most basic fashion, breast surgery treats disease by removing breast tissue. However, in reality there are many different ways in which breast disease is treated by surgery, with variable outcomes in the appearance of a woman's breast following treatment (surgery).

When you are faced with the recommendation of breast surgery to treat disease, you must ask several very specific questions:

- Is the purpose of the proposed surgery to diagnose disease? To treat disease? Or both?
- Is surgery the only form of treatment necessary?
- What are the likely physical outcomes to my health and appearance resulting from the recommended surgery?
- What alternatives do I have?
- What are my rights regarding the alternatives?

Once you have answers to these questions, you likely will find yourself with many more questions. Among those questions, you must define a plan for your goals, and then enlist the medical specialists you need prior to any surgery to treat your breast disease and achieve realistic goals for your health and your appearance.

The key medical specialists to consult are a general or breast surgeon and a board-certified plastic surgeon.

- The breast surgeon will likely perform your breast surgery specific to treating disease

- The plastic surgeon will partner or consult with your breast surgeon in any surgery you undergo, so that you may benefit from reconstruction at the time of surgery to treat disease, or other surgery that is planned for the future

But your agenda does not end with enlisting the right providers for your care: You must now pre-certify your breast surgery with your insurance company. During what may be a highly stressful time for you, insurers may, in fact, not be the most cooperative. They will likely require ample paperwork from any physician who you consult with or who will treat you. Take charge of administering exactly what they require in the same fashion you have taken charge of who will perform your breast surgery. You must be proactive. It is up to you to discover what is needed from each party and make sure that all of the insurance paperwork has been received from the physician's office. Keeping good lines of communication open will maintain the momentum of this process.

Although many forms of breast reconstruction and reconstruction in general are discussed in this section, refer to Part VI: Breast Reconstruction for detailed information on breast reconstruction procedures and issues.

According to the National Institutes of Health and the National Cancer Institute, in 2004 approximately 140,000 women were diagnosed with breast cancer, two-thirds of which will be localized and will not have spread beyond the tumor in the breast. For more information and related statistics, visit *www.nci.nih.gov.*

41. Is breast surgery used strictly to treat breast cancer?

No, breast surgery treats much more than breast cancer. Research data from the Institute of Medicine and the National Institutes of Health (NIH) state that roughly 80% of all breast lumps are **benign** (harmless), and some may be treated with surgery. These include benign cysts, tumors, and calcification. Additionally, breast surgery can treat blocked and infected milk ducts, and can also treat medical conditions that result from excessively heavy and large breasts, such as back and neck pain, breast pain, rashes and skin ulcers (see Part VII: Breast Reduction; Questions 65–72).

42. What is a lumpectomy or breast conserving surgery?

In some cases of tumor removal, including breast cancer, a **lumpectomy**, or breast conserving surgery may be prescribed. Lumpectomy means that only a portion of the breast is removed: the tumor and a small area of the surrounding healthy tissue (**margin**). With lumpectomy, as much healthy breast tissue as possible will be conserved. The goal of lumpectomy is minimal disfigurement and effective treatment. However, this does not mean that the procedure will not cause you any disfigurement. A lumpectomy can result in changes to breast size and shape.

When a lumpectomy is followed by radiation, this is considered **breast conserving surgery** and is an alternative in some cases for a mastectomy (which is the complete removal of the breast). This is most often recommended when a breast tumor is considered to be

Benign

a nonmalignant neoplasm or mild character of an illness.

Lumpectomy

type of surgical removal of a tumor involving breast conserving surgery.

Margin

area of healthy tissue surrounding a tumor, cyst, or calcification; surgically removed with the lump to make certain all of the abnormal tissue cells are included.

Breast conserving surgery

lumpectomy is followed by radiation; considered an alternative in some cases for a mastectomy.

invasive breast cancer, meaning that the cancer is outside the confines of the milk ducts, or for certain types of in situ breast cancer (cancer contained within the ducts). The added radiation can cause skin discoloration in addition to the change in breast size or shape.

If your goals are to look and feel whole again following any ablative breast surgery (removal of the breast), including lumpectomy, you should consult with a breast surgeon to determine if consultations with a plastic surgeon prior to the surgery to treat disease is warranted. Both will work together to provide you the best possible outcomes for your health, and for reconstruction if it is likely to be prescribed.

A wide excision biopsy or **quadrantectomy** is sometimes confused for lumpectomy. These procedures do remove localized breast tissue. However, the wide excision biopsy is more often for diagnostic goals that may result in full or partial removal of possibly malignant tumors. A quadrantectomy is removal of one quarter or quadrant of the breast, and can be highly disfiguring.

43. How is a lumpectomy performed?

Lumpectomy is performed by removing a breast tumor or cancer, and also removing a margin of healthy tissue surrounding the tumor. Additional tissue will continue to be removed in that initial surgical session until the surgeon arrives at what is called a **"clear" margin**, or area around the tumor that shows no preliminary evidence of cancer. Following surgery, a complete microscopic evaluation is done of the outermost margin of healthy tissue. If tumor cells are found to be present at

Invasive breast cancer

when cancer cells migrate to tissues outside of the confines of the milk ducts.

In situ breast cancer

when cancer cells are contained within the milk ducts.

Quadrantectomy

a wide excision biopsy involving the removal of one quarter or quadrant of the breast; can be highly disfiguring.

Clear margin

area around a tumor that shows no preliminary evidence of cancerous cells.

Treating Breast Disease

this stage of evaluation, then further surgery, or a re-excision, will likely be recommended so that additional tissue and all possible cancerous cells are removed. Depending on the extent of the re-excision necessary, a mastectomy may be recommended.

Good Candidates

Good candidates for lumpectomy are generally women who have no previous history of breast cancer in the affected breast, or fewer than two current areas of beast cancer in the same breast. In addition, good candidates have not previously had radiation to the chest or afflicted breast area.

Women who are pregnant and whose cancers will likely require localized radiation may not be good candidates for breast conserving surgery, as added radiation therapy may harm the fetus. In addition, women who are not good candidates for radiation therapy because of other medical conditions, like connective tissue disorders (CTD), are not good candidates for breast conserving surgery. In cases where tumors are located in aesthetically sensitive areas, such as directly behind the nipple and areola, a mastectomy may be recommended because a lumpectomy can be highly disfiguring.

In general, women with tumors estimated to be 5 centimeters in diameter or larger, or small-breasted women whose tumors are large in relation to breast size, may not be good candidates for lumpectomy, as it is more likely the procedure will be highly disfiguring.

The Surgery Experience

Depending on the extent of your lumpectomy and your overall health, the procedure may be performed on an outpatient basis using local anesthetic with or without sedation, or with a general anesthesia. An in-patient hospital stay may also be recommended, particularly if the disfigurement is significant enough to require reconstruction.

Most cases of lumpectomy do not require formal breast reconstruction. Occasionally, a local rearrangement of remaining breast tissue at the time of lumpectomy can minimize a deformity caused by removing breast tissue. If formal reconstruction using the woman's own tissue moved from another part of the body to the breast is recommended, this is usually delayed. Reconstruction will take place after pathological confirmation of **negative margins** (no additional malignant cells in tissue surrounding the tumor) or after the final extent of the deformity has been ascertained.

Following Surgery

Surgery performed on an outpatient basis allows you to recover at home, barring any complication or unexpected events during surgery. Inpatient surgery, with or without reconstruction, will include a one- to two-night hospital stay. However, a flap procedure for reconstruction may extend your stay to three to five days or more (see Questions 56–60). You will likely experience localized swelling and tenderness in your breast. Your pain and discomfort will likely be localized to the area where surgery was performed on the breast, and can be comfortably controlled with medication.

As healing progresses, you may notice your incision sites are firm and may become somewhat itchy. It is important to follow your surgeon's advice with regard to cleansing wounds, leaving surgical tape intact, and applying ointments as recommended. This will help the scars to heal. In addition, a soft

Negative margins
no additional malignant cells are in tissue surrounding the tumor.

Treating Breast Disease

support bra (without underwires) or camisole with a shelf bra may be most comfortable in those first few days. Avoid anything that applies too much pressure to the breast.

Drains

medical tubing placed in wound cavities to remove fluid.

Lumpectomy does not generally require **drains** at the surgical site, but in some cases they may be used. Drains are hollow tubes placed in a wound cavity to prevent fluid collection. If drains are used, they will be removed within several days following surgery, depending upon the recommendation of your breast surgeon.

Cautions and Considerations

Risks of lumpectomy include potential risks following any surgery, and are fully discussed in Question #19. In addition, there is the possibility of a developing a **seroma** (fluid collection in the space where the tumor was removed) that does not resolve. This can generally be drained though **aspiration** (removal with a needle) in your surgeon's office. Although rare, the space may continue to collect fluid. If this happens, treatment includes compression to close the space.

Seroma

fluid collection in the space where tissue was removed.

Aspiration

removal of fluid collected inside a body cavity with a needle.

While there is a high success rate with lumpectomy and breast conserving surgery, immediate reconstruction with the use of a breast implant is generally not recommended in these cases. Mammography and follow-up to carefully monitor any recurrence of the tumor or cancer is essential to your course of treatment and, depending on the location of the original cancer or tumor, a breast implant may interfere with the ability to detect some changes in the breast tissue through mammography.

Back to Life

In general, women who undergo lumpectomy may be back to moderate activity within a day or two of returning home. Within two weeks, most women are fully active, although the necessary radiation treatments with breast conserving surgery may have some side effects that slow you down.

Lumpectomy is a procedure that is growing in numbers, due to the success of outcomes both in your health, and in the appearance of your breast. Careful planning with your breast surgeon and plastic surgeon, and a review of all your options is essential to your satisfaction and your overall health prognosis.

While the physical stress of lumpectomy may be much less than a mastectomy, you still need time to recuperate, both physically and emotionally. The support of your family and friends may not be enough. Ask your surgeon or physician for local support groups or sources of individual support in your area to give you the assistance you need to get back to your daily life.

According to an October 2002 study published in the *New England Journal of Medicine*, women treated with lumpectomy and radiation were as likely to be alive and disease free 20 years after surgery as those women who had radical mastectomy. The National Cancer Institutes stated, "Long-term survival is identical with breast conserving surgery and radiation therapy, compared with mastectomy."

44. What is a mastectomy?

Mastectomy

complete surgical removal of the breast, most often including the nipple/areola complex. A simple or total mastectomy includes all breast tissue, down to, but not including, the chest wall muscle or the lymph glands. The result is the complete absence of a breast on the chest wall, with a horizontal scar where the breast was once located.

Modified radical mastectomy

a type of mastectomy that includes the removal of the axillary (underarm) lymph nodes.

Radical mastectomy

a type of mastectomy that is performed only in extreme cases, which includes the removal of the major and minor pectoral (chest) muscles.

A **mastectomy** is generally defined as the complete surgical removal of the breast, most often including the nipple/areola complex. A simple or total mastectomy includes all breast tissue, down to, but not including, the chest wall muscle. It may or may not include removal of the nipple/areola complex. It does not include removal of the lymph glands. The result is the complete absence of a breast on the chest wall, with a horizontal scar where the breast was once located.

A **modified radical mastectomy** is a total mastectomy with removal of the axillary (underarm) lymph nodes. A **radical mastectomy**, performed only in extreme cases, also includes removal of the major and minor pectoral (chest) muscles.

There are also more minor procedures sometimes categorized as mastectomy. These include: a quadrantectomy, where a quarter or defined section of the breast skin and all soft tissue is removed, often including local lymph nodes; and a **partial or segmental mastectomy**, where a larger segment of the breast than in a lumpectomy is removed, but some of the breast tissue and skin is preserved, and, in limited cases, this may include the nipple/areola complex.

In addition, skin-sparing mastectomy has recently become a very positive alternative to a standard mastectomy and is fully discussed in Question 46.

45. How is a mastectomy performed?

A mastectomy is major surgery and should always be performed in a hospital setting under general anesthesia. Your doctor will likely recommend a short hospital stay following your mastectomy. The reasons for an in-patient stay include the need for both a physical and emotional recuperation following mastectomy. You will likely have drainage tubes for several days following surgery, and require careful monitoring for pain management and any immediate complications. At the time this book was written, the Breast Cancer Patient Protection Act of 2004 was pending, requiring insurers in the United States to allow coverage for a minimum two-night hospital stay following a mastectomy. Senator Mary Landrieu (D-LA) and Representative Rosa DeLauro (D-CT) will reintroduce this act in Congress in 2005 bi-partisan legislation to end this practice. This petition, driven by *Lifetimetv.com*, is a partnership with physicians, advocates, and survivors across the nation.

Mastectomy completely removes the breast, but immediate reconstruction is possible for most candidates at the time of mastectomy, including:

- Any one of several flap surgery techniques
- Tissue expansion and the subsequent placement of a breast implant

If you are considering immediate reconstruction, your breast surgeon and plastic surgeon should both be consulted prior to surgery, and should communicate with one another.

However, due to additional treatments and therapies, or to your current health condition, a delayed reconstruction may be recommended. In this case, for the

Partial or segmental mastectomy

a type of mastectomy where a larger segment of the breast than in a lumpectomy is surgically removed, but some of the breast tissue and skin are preserved, and, in limited cases, the nipple/areola complex are also preserved.

Treating Breast Disease

best possible aesthetic outcomes, you still should consult with both surgeons prior to your mastectomy and have the surgeons consult with one another. Your plastic surgeon may have specific recommendations for your mastectomy with regard to incision patterns and the resulting scar placement that could greatly influence the results of your reconstruction.

If you have decided to delay reconstruction yourself, or are uncertain about your decision for reconstruction, it is still advised that you consult with a plastic surgeon about your options. What you learn during your consultation may, in fact, help you to make your reconstruction decision. You certainly may make the choice to forgo reconstruction; it is your choice.

Good Candidates

The same candidates for breast conserving surgery (lumpectomy and subsequent localized radiation therapy) may also be candidates for mastectomy. Mastectomy will most likely be recommended if: cancer has recurred following lumpectomy; cancer is present in more than one area of the breast; the cancer is particularly invasive, depending on the stage of cancer diagnosed and based on your own breast health history and your family breast health history; or if a lumpectomy will result in an aesthetically unacceptable breast.

Nearly all mastectomy candidates are candidates for breast reconstruction. Even women with high risk factors such as diabetes, connective tissue disorders, or heavy smokers, have the potential for reconstruction if the health conditions or behaviors that may impair healing can be controlled or eliminated.

Good candidates for **immediate reconstruction** (reconstruction performed at the time of mastectomy) are women whose subsequent course of cancer treatment (radiation to the chest area or chemotherapy) will not interfere with healing, and who are otherwise in good health and able to withstand the additional surgery. In addition, women who are having emotional difficulty facing their diagnosis and prescribed course of treatment may be advised to first manage their health, and then weigh reconstructive options once they feel strong enough to undergo surgery again.

Immediate reconstruction

breast reconstruction performed at the time of mastectomy.

Surgery Experience

Mastectomy is an inpatient hospital procedure performed under general anesthesia. It is major surgery lasting from two to three hours if immediate reconstruction is not planned, and requires a team of medical professionals who include: your surgeon or surgeons, an anesthesiologist, and a team of nurses or surgical assistants.

An incision is made on the breast, and underlying fat, tissue, and glands are **excised** (separated from the surrounding tissues and removed). Even if the nipple/areola is not removed, the mammary glands and surrounding nerves are detached from the nipple and removed. After mastectomy, if the nipple is preserved, sensation to the nipple is minimal, and normal breastfeeding is not possible. Once the breast tissue has been removed, any remaining skin is sutured together or closed with temporary metal clips. A slightly curved

Excised

fat, tissue, and glands are separated from the surrounding tissues and removed.

Treating Breast Disease

and slightly angled horizontal incision will remain across the chest where the breast once was positioned. The incisions may, however, vary and if you have any consideration of future reconstruction, it is best to have your plastic surgeon consult with the breast surgeon on mastectomy incisions and resulting scar location.

If you are having immediate reconstruction, your surgery may be extended by one or several hours. Part 6 (Questions 50–64) details all breast reconstruction options, and considerations for immediate reconstruction following mastectomy are addressed in Questions 53 and 54.

During closure for mastectomy or mastectomy with immediate reconstruction, small flexible tubes are likely to be placed from your incisions to drain any excess fluid that accumulates.

Following Surgery

Don't think you will feel like yourself. You will cry. You will be angry. And there will be times that you will be hopeful for the future. The support of those you love, and new friends that you meet in support groups, are essential to your experience before and following surgery. There are always those good-intentioned friends and relatives who want to help that you would rather not have around. Don't feel you have to accept the help of everyone, and especially those with whom you cannot share your emotions. Take and ask for help from those you want. And there is nothing wrong with politely declining help from those with whom you just don't have complete comfort. If they really care about you and your feelings, they will understand and give you the space and time you need.

—Ann

Your surgical stay following mastectomy may range from two days to as many as eight days or more, depending on: your surgery; your overall health; the recommendations of your surgeon or surgeons; whether or not you had immediate reconstruction or any subsequent treatments; and what your insurer will allow.

You will experience discomfort in the first few days following surgery in the chest area in general and in any donor sites if you have had immediate reconstruction. Oral medication and a pain pump can help control your discomfort. In addition, you may experience some swelling in the arm and chest, and in any donor sites if you have had immediate flap reconstruction. Some patients experience discomfort raising their arms, or a pulling sensation in the chest region. This is particularly true of radical mastectomy and if the axillary (underarm) lymph glands were also removed.

Drainage tubes may be removed within a few days or a week or more following your surgery. In addition, before being released from the hospital, you will be given detailed instructions for wound care and cleansing. Other instructions will include: activity restrictions and suggestions; proper diet and required exercise; when you may resume wearing a bra and what type to wear; and if you have not had reconstruction when you may begin wearing a prosthesis. In addition, you will be given medications for pain and to prevent infection, be instructed about specific changes to look for in the surgical site and your overall health, and when these require you to contact your surgeon.

Cautions and Considerations

Cautions following mastectomy are like those of any breast surgery, and are defined in Question 19. In addition, it is not uncommon for women to have sensations following mastectomy with or without immediate reconstruction, such as itching, nerve impulses or numbness, pressure, and throbbing. Report any of these feelings to your surgeon immediately, as there are treatment options to alleviate these often uncomfortable experiences.

You will be given specific instructions with regard to resuming normal activity and exercise. Follow these instructions carefully. While getting back to life is an important part of your physical and emotional recovery, to do so too soon, or too strenuously, can compromise your health and cause bleeding, tearing of healing skin and tissue, and even orthopedic injury to adjacent muscles.

Back to Life

Depending on your overall health, additional treatments recommended, the extent of your mastectomy, and if you have had immediate reconstruction, you can plan on getting back to a moderate pace of activity within two to three weeks following your surgery. If you have had immediate reconstruction, you will likely follow up with your breast surgeon and your plastic surgeon. In addition to the support of your family and friends, ask your surgeon about special support groups and one-on-one sources of support from other breast cancer survivors and women who have undergone mastectomy. Your physical rehabilitation is very important. Equally important is your need for emotional support and healing. If you have not had recon-struction, but are considering it, you may follow up with your plastic surgeon when you feel ready.

According to the American Society of Plastic Surgeons, breast reconstruction procedures numbered nearly 62,930 in 2004. That is a slow and steady decline over recent years. The likely cause is an increase in the number of lumpectomies for small tumors and a decrease in the number of mastectomies.

46. What is a skin-sparing mastectomy?

A skin-sparing mastectomy is a refined technique that allows women who choose immediate reconstruction some of the best possible aesthetic outcomes. This requires the plastic surgeon to guide the breast surgeon in incision patterns for the mastectomy. These are typi-cally in a concentric pattern around the nipple/areola complex, and may possibly extend vertically from the bottom of the areola to just above the breast crease or laterally from the side of the areola toward the axilla (underarm). The breast or cancer surgeon then removes the underlying tissue leaving the overlying skin intact. The nipple and areola may or may not be removed.

The plastic surgeon then performs the immediate reconstruction. This is done using a flap from the abdomen, back, buttock, or thigh to provide the tissue bulk needed to reconstruct the breast. For thin women who may not be ideal candidates for flap surgery, skin-sparing mastectomy with immediate reconstruction using a breast implant provides a good option. For nearly all women, it reduces the visible scars on the breast, and provides some of the most pleasing aes-thetic outcomes.

47. Can I choose between a lumpectomy, skin-sparing mastectomy, or mastectomy?

Patient selection is the key in determining whether lumpectomy, skin-sparing mastectomy, or mastectomy is best for you. Two key factors in patient selection include:

- The size, location, and type of tumor or cancer present, and the best possible treatment to ensure your health
- The cosmetic result of certain procedures and your desire for reconstruction

If your goals reach beyond treating your breast disease, the cosmetic result of your procedure and any plan for reconstruction require the cooperation and involvement of your breast surgeon, oncologist, and your plastic surgeon. Your health must be the primary factor in determining any form of treatment. You may, in fact, be given the choice of procedures. Make your decision based on your personal goals for health, your personal and realistic goals for reconstruction, and the advice of your plastic surgeon. Plastic surgeons who are experienced in breast reconstruction work closely with breast cancer surgeons. They fully understand and uphold your health considerations before making a prescription for reconstruction.

Preventative (or prophylactic) mastectomy

the removal of one or both breasts to prevent breast cancer from developing in a woman with a family history of breast cancer or to reduce a woman's chance of developing breast cancer.

48. Is mastectomy always performed to treat disease?

There are women who elect to undergo mastectomy as a means to prevent breast cancer. **Preventative (or prophylactic) mastectomy** is the removal of one or both breasts to prevent breast cancer from developing or to reduce a woman's chance of developing breast cancer.

Reasons why a woman may choose preventative mastectomy, or have the procedure recommended to her, include:

- A strong family history of breast cancer, namely, those forms of breast cancer known to be hereditary traits or where close relatives have died from breast cancer before the age of 50
- A positive test that demonstrates the woman carries the *BRCA1* or *BRCA2* genes
- An invasive form of breast cancer on the opposite breast
- Prior invasive forms of cancer near the breast area or in the axilla (underarm area)
- A very large number of breast calcifications and very dense breast tissue

A preventative mastectomy can reduce a woman's chances of developing breast cancer, but nothing can completely eliminate the risk for breast cancer.

Preventative mastectomy does offer additional advantages. Preventative mastectomy allows a woman to plan for her surgery. With ample time to plan, she may feel less stressed, and therefore have plenty of time to learn about and weigh her reconstructive options.

There are alternatives to preventative mastectomy, and these should be carefully discussed with your personal physician and a cancer specialist. These include: medications such as tamoxifen; close monitoring of breast health and changes by the woman and her physician; and potential alterations in diet, alcohol consumption, and tobacco use. The use of hormone replacement therapy and its role in the development of breast cancer is highly controversial, and should be discussed with your personal physician or cancer specialist. To date, no studies reveal whether preventative mastectomy or any of the available alternatives offer higher success rates and satisfaction for women who are at high risk for developing breast cancer.

It is important to understand that prophylactic mastectomy is a very serious decision. The outcomes are permanent, there is no guarantee that you will not develop any form of cancer, and the reconstructed breast will never be the same as the natural breast.

A study published in the January 14, 1999 issue of the *New England Journal of Medicine* was based on a retrospective study of 693 women who had prophylactic mastectomies between 1960 and 1993 at the Mayo Clinic. The study concluded that in women with a high risk of developing breast cancer, prophylactic mastectomy was associated with a reduction in the incidence of breast cancer of at least 90%.

49. What are my rights for insurance coverage for breast surgery to treat disease?

Insurers in the United States are mandated to provide coverage for ablative breast surgery, breast reconstruction, and for additional procedures prescribed for the opposite breast necessary for achieving symmetry.

Today any woman who undergoes mastectomy is entitled to coverage for reconstruction by her insurer. In addition, most women do not know—and often are not told—that insurance companies are required by law to cover *any* procedures of breast reconstruction. In the United States, this is the result of the 1998 Federal Breast Reconstruction Law. The enactment of this law is directly a result of the patient advocacy efforts led by the American Society of Plastic Surgeons.

Specifically, the law defines that if your insurer covers breast surgery to treat or prevent disease, you have the legal right to equal insurance coverage to consult with a plastic surgeon and have him or her fully involved in your case. You may be limited to providers based on your plan, and there may be pre-certification requirements including the need for a referral from your family physician or breast surgeon. But your insurance must cover prescribed ablative breast surgery and it must provide equal coverage for reconstruction and the services of a board-certified plastic surgeon to:

- Consult in your case
- Participate in your surgery
- Perform any resulting reconstruction prescribed by that plastic surgeon

Coverage does not end here. The same law includes coverage rights for procedures determined by your plastic surgeon to achieve symmetry between both breasts following ablative breast surgery. These procedures may include a breast reduction, breast lift, or breast augmentation.

You must know your rights with regard to your health and your body. The decision of what type of reconstruction to have is one to be made together with your plastic surgeon, and not to be dictated by your insurer. To have those rights met will likely require pre-certification. Both your breast surgeon's and your plastic surgeon's offices will provide the documentation necessary for coverage or assist you in filing for insurance coverage. However, these are *your* rights. Despite the cooperation and administrative management of your surgeon's office related to your case and coverage, either you or a close and trusted family member, someone who has defined rights to your health care information and management, must closely monitor insurance issues and keep records of all documents and communications related to coverage.

The day I was diagnosed with breast cancer, I began two journals: one about my feelings and one to document my experiences, managing the case from an education and administrative standpoint. When the bills and insurance denials from my mastectomy and my reconstruction arrived, having that second journal was imperative. It helped me to keep a record of conversations and correspondence, and made the job of dealing with my insurer a lot more organized and less stressful.

—Ann

You can obtain the exact text of the 1998 Federal Breast Reconstruction Law and a state-by-state update of laws related to breast reconstruction at *www.plasticsurgery.org.*

PART SIX

Breast Reconstruction

What is breast reconstruction?

Who is a good candidate for breast reconstruction?

Who performs breast reconstruction?

More . . .

50. What is breast reconstruction?

Breast reconstruction is surgery to restore the physical appearance of a breast resulting most often from acquired deformities. Acquired deformities are those where a breast has been completely lost or disfigured as the result of breast surgery to treat breast disease, or trauma.

The origins of breast reconstruction date back to the 1890s and documentation of attempts to use early surgical techniques to rebuild a breast from a flap (where skin, fat, and other tissue is transplanted from one part of the body to another). It was not until the later part of the 1900s, however, that breast reconstruction became a very specific focus of plastic surgery. Advancements in surgery resulted in the advent of flaps to cover and support a breast implant in the 1970s. Then, in 1982, the first completely reconstructed breast using a woman's own tissue taken from her abdomen, called a **TRAM (transverse rectus abdominus musculocutaneous)** flap, was performed. Currently, through the use of **microsurgery** (the reattachment of nerves and vessels in surgery performed via microscope and microsurgical techniques), breast reconstruction can be accomplished with a woman's own tissue while minimizing functional problems from the site of the donor tissue.

The use of breast implants and microsurgery and flap techniques remain the basis for all breast reconstructions today. Refinements are continuously evolving and allow for reconstructed breasts that are remarkably natural looking and feel very natural to the touch as well. However, much like nature is not always perfect, surgery to mimic nature does not result in the perfect replacement of a woman's natural breast. All

Breast reconstruction

a type of surgery to restore the physical appearance of a breast resulting most often from acquired deformities; acquired deformities are those where a breast has been completely lost or disfigured as the result of breast surgery to treat breast disease, or trauma.

TRAM (transverse rectus abdominus musculocutaneous)

type of breast surgery where a flap using a woman's own tissue taken from her abdomen is used to reconstruct a breast.

Microsurgery

where the reattachment of nerves and vessels in surgery is performed via microscope and microsized surgical tools.

cases of breast reconstruction will leave some visible scarring on or near the breast. Reconstruction of the nipple and areola can look highly natural; however, it will not have the same sensation of a natural nipple. No woman with a completely reconstructed breast can breast-feed naturally, as the mammary glands have been removed. And, a reconstructed breast may not match the shape and slope of the breast it replaces. Breast reconstruction allows a woman to have a positive self-image, feeling confident of her body and herself in her most public and intimate encounters in life.

You may be thankful for your health, and you may be angry about losing a breast or having one that is disfigured. Breast reconstruction is amazing. It may not be perfect, but the result is one that I have actively lived with confidently for several years. I wear just about anything I want. I swim, I play tennis, and I can hold my husband and my children close without feeling like a part of me is missing. Even if you don't believe you want reconstruction, learn about it. You may find yourself feeling one day that you deserve to have a breast that is a part of your body.

—Ann

The National Institutes of Health reported that nearly 165,000 women were diagnosed with breast cancer in 2000. That same year, over 80,000 breast reconstruction procedures were performed. The assumption is that somewhat less than half of all women who are diagnosed with breast cancer will undergo reconstruction. However, of those diagnosed, there are missing data, including the number of those with mastectomy versus lumpectomy (also called breast conserving surgery [BCR]).

At present we do not have statistics that define how many women diagnosed with breast cancer received information about breast reconstruction. Some studies estimate that as many as one third to one half of women who undergo some form of surgery to remove a portion of or a complete breast due to disease do not receive any information about reconstruction.

51. Who is a good candidate for breast reconstruction?

Good candidates for surgical breast reconstruction are determined by four factors:

- Individual desire: You want to look and feel whole with a breast that is part of your own body.
- Physician recommendations: Your surgeon or plastic surgeon recommends or prescribes breast reconstruction to address your individual circumstances and your desire.
- Timing: When reconstruction is medically appropriate and when you feel ready to invest the time necessary for surgery and to heal.
- General health: When the state of your overall health does not put you at added risk for complications.

Nearly all women with acquired deformities of the breast are good candidates for breast reconstruction. The exception is any health condition that can greatly impair a woman's ability to heal or increase her risk of very serious complications during or following surgery. In addition, timing can define good candidates for breast reconstruction. In some cases, a woman undergoing or who will undergo certain medical treatments in the future (such as chemotherapy or radiation therapy) may not be a good candidate to have breast reconstruction until those treatments are completed. Additionally, a woman who is uncertain of her personal goals, has unrealistic expectations for breast reconstruction, or who is unable to confidently make a decision about breast reconstruction, may be not be a good candidate. Women who are having emotional difficulty dealing with a diagnosis of breast disease and ablative surgery may be advised to get emotional support before making a decision about breast reconstruction.

According to the American Society of Plastic Surgeons, breast reconstruction procedures numbered nearly 62,930 in 2004, and show a slow and steady decline over recent years. The likely cause is an increase in the number of lumpectomies for small tumors and a decrease in the number of mastectomies.

52. Who performs breast reconstruction?

Breast reconstruction is performed by board-certified plastic surgeons. Breast reconstruction is a **plastic surgery** procedure, with plastic surgery being the defined specialty of medicine that includes training specific to the techniques and procedures that rebuild a woman's breast.

Breast reconstruction may also be defined as a reconstructive procedure among plastic surgery procedures. However, there is no defined specialty of reconstructive surgery, nor is there a defined subspecialty of reconstructive surgery. There is nothing that prevents other medical or surgical specialists from performing breast reconstruction; however, the only specialty with defined training in breast reconstruction is plastic surgery.

Plastic surgery of the breast

any surgical procedure that changes or restores the appearance of the breast, including those procedures to treat and prevent breast disease that result in the change of a breast appearance.

53. When can breast reconstruction be performed?

The process of breast reconstruction can sometimes begin at the time of mastectomy or lumpectomy. Reconstruction may be delayed depending on additional prescribed medical treatments (chemotherapy or radiation therapy) based on the recommendation of your oncologist. It may also be delayed if that is your preference.

Dealing with breast cancer or tumor removal is a very difficult process. The ability to awaken from any ablative breast surgery (which is surgery that removes all or a portion of the breast) with the beginnings of a new breast mound already in place can be immensely important to a woman. But you cannot pursue immediate reconstruction if you don't discuss your options for reconstruction with your surgeon and with a plastic surgeon before ablative breast surgery.

Immediate reconstruction offers a woman the advantage of sparing her from the experience of completely losing a breast or seeing herself severely disfigured. It also spares a woman subsequent major surgery. As well, the outcomes of breast reconstruction can be somewhat enhanced when the surgeon performing your ablative breast surgery and your plastic surgeon can work together through such things as skin-sparing techniques and optimal incision placement.

The greatest benefit of immediate reconstruction is that it may allow you to feel whole again and return to your normal life more quickly. As a result, your emotional and physical health will benefit greatly. But if you cannot undergo immediate reconstruction, knowing your options will give you some encouragement for your future ability to feel whole. Therefore, it is important to consider breast reconstruction and all of your options before undergoing ablative breast surgery. Discuss this with your surgeon, and consult with a plastic surgeon as soon as possible.

54. Can I undergo cancer treatments during or following reconstruction?

Every case of breast cancer is highly individual. There are some standards; but every standard has exceptions. Therefore, you must consult with your surgeon, your oncologist, and your plastic surgeon in every case. In cases where your breast cancer is more advanced, or depending on the type of cancer diagnosed, you may be advised to undergo radiation therapy or chemotherapy in addition to ablative breast surgery.

Radiation Therapy

In general, women who will undergo radiation may have immediate reconstruction. However, radiation may not likely begin until healing has progressed. It is important to understand that radiation may cause changes to skin that may potentially distort the natural or reconstructed breast tissue. Therefore, to delay reconstruction following radiation therapy may, in fact, limit your options in reconstruction, such as tissue expansion and subsequent implant placement. However, radiation after immediate reconstruction may damage the reconstructed breast and require further surgery. Therefore, it is important that your oncologist and plastic surgeon consult prior to any surgery, and the pros and cons of immediate and/or delayed reconstruction be fully discussed relative to any planned radiation.

Chemotherapy

Women who will undergo chemotherapy may be advised to delay reconstruction depending on the extent of the cancer and the woman's overall prognosis. However, immediate reconstruction is a safe option for many women who will also undergo chemotherapy, so long as chemotherapy may be delayed until initial wound healing has completed, which is generally three to four weeks following surgery.

A 2001 study published in the *Plastic and Reconstructive Surgery Journal* stated that patients who underwent immediate flap reconstruction and subsequent chemotherapy experienced similar complications and delays to post-operative chemotherapy as patients who delayed reconstruction. The most common reason for postponement of chemotherapy following reconstruction or mastectomy was waiting for the wound to heal. Delays in chemotherapy treatment were defined to average three weeks, and the delays did not have significant impact on the effectiveness of chemotherapy treatments.

The National Cancer Institute offers the latest standards in breast cancer treatment on their Web site, *www.nci.nih.gov*, with links to "breast cancer" and then to "treatment" and "patients."

55. What are my options for breast reconstruction?

Learn about all of the options, even if they are not all appropriate for you. It helps you to understand the differences between them and to better understand why your surgeon and plastic surgeon recommend a specific reconstruction technique for you.

There are four general options in breast reconstruction techniques, or surgery to rebuild the breast mound. Not all of these options may be appropriate for you.

- The use of a breast implant, often in conjunction with a technique called tissue expansion (see Question 56).
- A **latissimus dorsi flap**, using a woman's own muscle, fat, and skin from her back. This is most often used to support a breast implant where little tissue remains at the chest wall to support and cover the implant (see Question 58). In a minor percentage of cases, this flap alone may be used to reconstruct the breast.
- A **pedicled TRAM** or transverse rectus abdominus musculocutaneous flap, using a woman's own muscle, fat, and skin from her abdomen. A pedicled TRAM flap remains tethered to its original blood supply (see Question 59).
- A **free flap**, using a woman's own, muscle, fat and skin from the abdomen, buttocks or thigh, transplanted to the chest wall, using microsurgical techniques (see Question 60).

All of these procedures result in creation of the breast mound, and all can be used in immediate reconstruction, although tissue expansion requires time before the complete breast mound has been formed. Creation of a nipple requires an additional procedure or procedures and is typically achieved using local flap, grafting, and/or tattooing techniques.

Determining what procedure is right for you is highly individualized based on your degree of deformity, the condition of any remaining breast tissue, your physical

Latissimus dorsi flap

a type of reconstruction surgery using a woman's own muscle, fat, and skin from her back; most often used to support a breast implant where little tissue remains at the chest wall to support and cover the implant. In a minor percentage of cases, this flap alone may be used to reconstruct the breast.

Pedicled TRAM

transverse rectus abdominus musculocutaneous flap for a type of breast reconstruction; uses a woman's own muscle, fat, and skin from her abdomen; remains tethered to its original blood supply.

Free flap

a type of breast reconstruction that uses a woman's own muscle, fat, and skin from the abdomen, buttocks, or thigh, transplanted to the chest wall, using microsurgical techniques.

build, and your health. Your plastic surgeon will also take into consideration your personal preference and goals for reconstruction. You must accept that not all procedures for reconstruction are appropriate options in every case.

You must also understand that not all plastic surgeons perform all breast reconstruction techniques. For example, a minority of plastic surgeons perform free flaps for breast reconstruction. Therefore, it is important to know all the options, and if the plastic surgeon you consult with cannot address an option you feel you wish to consider or need more information about, ask for a referral to a plastic surgeon who can address these options.

56. What is tissue expansion?

Tissue expansion is a means to reconstruct the breast using a breast implant without a flap, where enough healthy skin and soft tissue necessary to cover an implant is not present. It involves the placement of an implant that is not completely filled, or of a tissue expander (a silicone shell balloon-like device) at the breast mound. Through gradual filling of the implant or expander over many weeks, enough healthy tissue is produced to cover a breast implant.

Good Candidates

Tissue expansion and placement of a breast implant is appropriate in most cases of unilateral (one side) or bilateral (both sides) breast reconstruction. However, women who have had prior radiation to the chest, or certain skin conditions or scarring may not be able to safely expand enough viable tissue to cover a breast implant. Because of changes in the skin that can result

Tissue expansion

a type of reconstruction of the breast using a breast implant, where enough healthy skin and soft tissue necessary to cover an implant is not present; involves the placement of an implant that is not completely filled, or of a tissue expander (a silicone shell balloon-like device) at the breast mound. Through gradual filling of the implant or expander over many weeks, enough healthy tissue is produced to cover a breast implant.

from radiation therapy, it is often not advised to undergo tissue expansion concurrently with radiation therapy. In addition, if you smoke, you may not be a good candidate for reconstruction of any kind and will likely be advised to quit smoking before any reconstructive procedure and for many weeks following surgery (see Question #22). To quit smoking for life is in the best interests of your health.

Surgery Experience

Tissue expansion begins with placement of a medical-grade, silicone shell balloon or a breast implant shell that over time is filled with sterile fluid through an internal, one-way valve. The implant shell may have a silicone outer form and a hollow inner cavity that allows tissue expansion, or it may be an unfilled saline breast implant.

Tissue expansion can begin an immediate reconstruction at the time of mastectomy, or be used in delayed reconstruction. In most cases, the procedure is performed under general anesthesia. Following tissue expansion at the time of ablative breast surgery, you will likely remain in the hospital for two or more days depending on the type of expander used and the degree of your ablative breast surgery. In some cases of delayed reconstruction, placement of the expander may be performed on an outpatient basis (Figure 1).

Following Surgery

Once your surgery is completed, you will likely be somewhat sore and experience discomfort in the chest area; this can be controlled with medication. In addition, you may notice a valve, or port from the implant

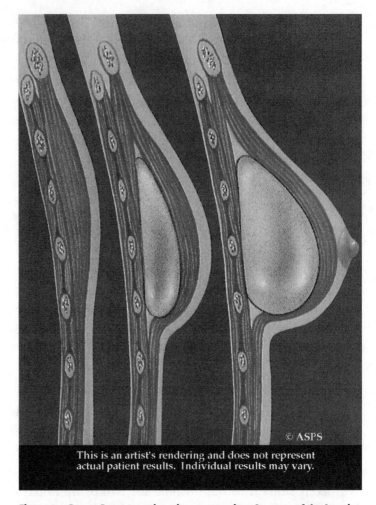

Figure 1   Breast Reconstruction: tissue expansion. Courtesy of the American Society of Plastic Surgeons®. All rights reserved. Learn more at www.plasticsurgery.org.

under your skin. This is where the implant will be filled with sterile fluid over time to achieve its final size. Initial discomfort should lessen significantly in the first three to four days following surgery. You should be ready for light, normal activity within three to four days following surgery.

Over the next few months or more, you will make several visits to your plastic surgeon's office to add fluid to the expander or implant. As the shell is filled and increases in size, it stretches the overlying skin and tissue. The goal of tissue expansion is to create enough healthy tissue to support a breast implant or to expand the implant to its final size. The process of tissue expansion is not one without discomfort. Each time more fluid is added, you will likely feel tightness in the chest region, and you may feel sore. It is important to discuss any discomfort with your plastic surgeon; prescription or over-the-counter medications will help make the tissue expansion a more comfortable process.

Once the process of tissue expansion is completed, the existing expander may be replaced with a final breast implant. Those expanders designed to serve as the final implant will be sealed, and any valve near the skin may be removed in a simple in-office procedure.

Cautions and Considerations

All of the complications and risks associated with breast surgery and with surgery in general are possible (see Question 19). Tissue expansion does require the use of a breast implant for your reconstruction and, therefore, all of the risks associated with the use of breast implants are possible (see Question 36).

Tissue expansion can result in areas of skin that are thinner or weaker, so the risk of implant extrusion (breaking through the skin surface) is somewhat higher. The best means to avoid this is to take all the time necessary for tissue expansion to achieve desired results, and avoid factors that can impair wound healing such as smoking.

Breast Reconstruction

115

Back to Life

Tissue expansion will not affect your daily routine; however, it may limit some of your exercise options. During the process of expansion, your figure will slowly evolve. Therefore, you may prefer to wear loose-fitting tops or padded bras to camouflage your evolving figure, or to softly pad a bra in order to lessen any asymmetry.

57. Does the use of a breast implant always require a flap or tissue expansion?

In most cases of mastectomy, there is not enough soft tissue remaining to cover an implant without significant risk of contracture, implant extrusion (breaking through the skin), or for a good result. However, some cases of skin-sparing mastectomy may retain enough skin and underlying soft tissue to allow for reconstruction with an implant and no additional procedures. Where lumpectomy or a partial mastectomy has significantly reduced breast size, the use of an implant without subsequent procedures may also be possible. However, if breast shape has been severely disfigured, a flap procedure and more advanced reconstruction may offer better outcomes.

In 2004, the American Society for Plastic Surgery (ASPS) reported over 16,424 breast implants used in breast reconstruction were surgically removed, of which 73% were replaced.

58. What is latissimus dorsi flap reconstruction?

The latissimus dorsi muscle is a long, flat muscle that runs diagonally from the side to midback. Reconstruction uses a flap of skin, soft tissue, and the latissimus muscle, which is relocated from the back to the breast region. However, unlike a TRAM that provides all the bulk necessary to create a breast mound, a **latissimus flap** has little fat and therefore is more often used to support and cover a breast implant in breast reconstruction.

Good Candidates

Most women are good candidates for a latissimus dorsi flap reconstruction. However, women who are very thin or who have pre-existing back or shoulder problems may not be good candidates for reconstruction with a latissimus dorsi flap. A latissimus dorsi flap may be performed bilaterally (on both sides).

Women who have chronic illnesses that may impair healing, such as diabetes or connective tissue disorders such as lupus, may not be good candidates for any breast reconstruction with flap surgery. In addition, if you smoke, you are not a good candidate for reconstruction of any kind and will be advised to quit smoking before any reconstructive procedure and for many weeks following. To quit smoking for life is in the best interests of your health (see Question 22).

Surgery Experience

A latissimus dorsi flap reconstruction is performed under general anesthesia as an inpatient hospital procedure. The procedure will add two or more hours if performed at the time of mastectomy, or may take several hours if delayed following mastectomy.

An elliptical incision in the back, just below the shoulder blade, is made. This allows your plastic surgeon to release the latissimus dorsi muscle from the midback

Breast Reconstruction

Latissimus flap
a type of breast reconstruction that uses a flap of skin, soft tissue, and the latissimus muscle, which is relocated from the back to the breast region. Unlike a TRAM that provides all the bulk necessary to create a breast mound, a latissimus flap has little fat and therefore is more often used to support and cover a breast implant in breast reconstruction.

and keep it attached to its original blood and nerve supply. A paddle of skin and tissue attached to the flap will remain in place. The flap is then rotated under the skin and soft tissue from the back to the front of the chest wall, in the region below the axilla (underarm). The muscle flap, tissue, and skin are positioned through the mastectomy incisions on the chest wall. The flap is fashioned to create a pocket for a breast implant using internal sutures. The implant is placed, and the resulting incisions on the back and breast mound are closed. Depending on your specific situation, your plastic surgeon may place a tissue expander behind the latissimus dorsi flap instead of placing a breast implant, and subsequently replace the tissue expander with a permanent breast implant in a future procedure (Figure 2).

Following Surgery

You will awaken from surgery with a full breast mound in place, if a permanent breast implant has been placed, or with a partial breast mound if an expander is used. Thin, flexible tubes may be placed in your incisions to drain any excess fluid that collects. You will experience discomfort, swelling, and tenderness at the new breast site and in your back where the flap was taken. Medication can be used to control your discomfort. In addition, you may experience a stiff and sore back, and find it difficult to lie on your back or lean back for a few days following surgery.

It is important to begin moving as instructed as soon as possible following surgery, to prevent blood clots from forming and to ease you into recovery. You will remain in the hospital for two to three days or more. Your release depends on your physical condition, the extent of the surgery, and your progress in healing.

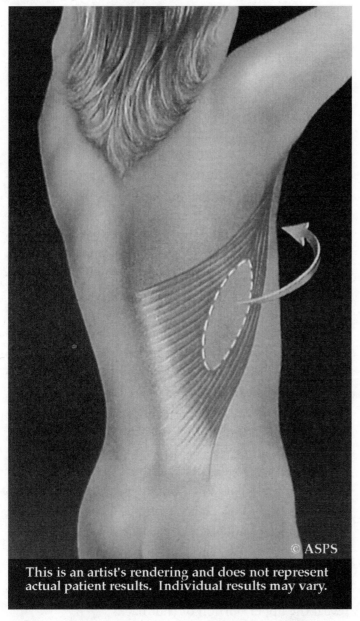

This is an artist's rendering and does not represent actual patient results. Individual results may vary.

Figure 2   Latissimus dorsi flap. Courtesy of the American Society of Plastic Surgeons®. All rights reserved. Learn more at *www.plasticsurgery.org*.

Cautions and Considerations

All of the complications and risks associated with breast surgery and with surgery in general are possible (see Question 19). In addition, if infection should develop and is not treated immediately you risk necrosis (pathologic death of one or more cells), of loss of the skin flap, and perhaps even surrounding healthy tissue.

Because a portion of your back muscle has been relocated, a latissimus dorsi flap procedure can result in an asymmetrical appearance of the back if performed unilaterally (on one side). In addition, weakness in the upper back is possible, as is developing shoulder pain because the muscles in the shoulder will compensate for any weakness in the mid- to upper-back.

A latissimus dorsi flap may allow for some physical sensation in the breast; however, it will take some time to develop or for you to recognize. In addition, because the flap is likely covering a breast implant, all of the risks associated with the use of breast implants are possible (see Question 36).

It is important to discuss incision placement on your back with your surgeon prior to your latissimus flap reconstruction. The incision on the back will leave a straight line scar that could measure 6 inches or more. In some cases, the scar may be placed to be hidden under the back portion of your bra, and low enough that you may feel comfortable wearing fashions that reveal the upper portion of your back.

Back to Life

Within two to four weeks following a latissimus dorsi flap reconstruction, you may be ready to get back to a moderate daily routine. Exercise is an important part of your recovery, but it is important to follow the instructions that you are given by your plastic surgeon or a physical therapist very closely. Too little exercise may hinder your recovery, and too much may result in unnecessary injury. It is important to maintain your back strength for life.

Although a latissimus dorsi flap itself does not hinder the methods used to monitor the reconstructed breast, continuous follow-ups as recommended by your surgeon, oncologist, and plastic surgeon are your best defense to leading a healthy life and feeling whole.

59. What is a pedicled TRAM flap reconstruction?

A pedicled TRAM (transverse rectus abdominus musculocutaneous) flap reconstructs a woman's breast using a flap of skin, fat, and muscle taken from a woman's lower abdomen, which is repositioned on the chest wall. The flap, or section of tissue taken from the lower abdomen, remains attached to the original blood supply. It is tunneled up to the breast mound site through the chest wall, and provides enough tissue to completely reconstruct the breast mound.

Good Candidates

Good candidates for a pedicled TRAM are women with sufficient healthy tissue in the abdominal region. Women who are very thin may not have sufficient tissue for an abdominal flap to fully reconstruct the breast. A pedicled TRAM may also not be appropriate in cases where a woman who has an excess of abdominal fat. In addition, women who have had previous abdominal surgeries where excess scar tissue remains, or where the abdominal wall is severely weakened, may not be good candidates for a pedicled TRAM reconstruction. Having enough abdominal tissue for a pedicled TRAM reconstruction is more common in unilateral (one side) cases of breast reconstruction, as fewer women have sufficient lower abdominal tissue to create two breast mounds.

Women who have chronic illnesses that may impair healing, such as diabetes or connective tissue disorders such as lupus, may not be good candidates for any breast reconstruction with flap surgery. In addition, if you smoke, you are not a good candidate for reconstruction of any kind and will be advised to quit smoking before any reconstructive procedure and for many weeks following. To quit smoking for life is in the best interests of your health (see Question 22).

Surgery Experience

A pedicled TRAM procedure is performed as an inpatient surgical procedure, under general anesthesia. It will add several hours to any ablative breast surgery, or may take several hours if performed in a delayed reconstruction. The procedure requires an elliptical incision pattern in the abdomen that is generally placed hip to hip at or below the bikini line. Through this incision, the underlying fat and muscle are separated from the abdominal wall. A paddle of skin and fat remains attached to the rectus abdominus muscle. The muscle is detached in the area of the bikini line incision, while the muscle above remains attached to the overlying skin and fat.

The muscle tether (with skin and fat attached) is tunneled up through the chest wall (below the skin, above the ribs) to either the opposite side from where it was detached or to the same side. It is brought up through the incisions where the breast has been removed or through new incisions to open the mastectomy site, depending upon whether the reconstruction is immediate or delayed. The muscle is shaped to form the underlying breast mound and fashioned with internal sutures, and the attached fat and skin are shaped to form the breast cushion and cover. The skin covering for the breast mound is shaped and incisions at the newly reconstructed beast site and in the abdomen are closed (Figure 3).

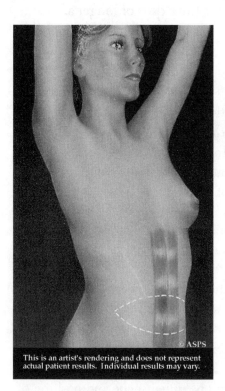

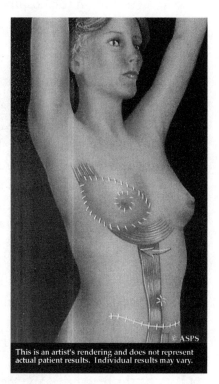

This is an artist's rendering and does not represent actual patient results. Individual results may vary.

This is an artist's rendering and does not represent actual patient results. Individual results may vary.

Figure 3 TRAM flap procedure. Courtesy of the American Society of Plastic Surgeons®. All rights reserved. Learn more at *www.plasticsurgery.org*.

Following Surgery

You will awaken from surgery with a full breast mound in place. Thin, flexible tubes may be placed in your incisions to drain any excess fluid that collects. You will experience discomfort, swelling, and tenderness at the new breast site and in the abdomen where the flap was taken. Medication can be used to control your discomfort. In addition, you may feel stiff and sore in the abdominal region and find it difficult to stand fully upright for a few days following surgery.

It is important to begin moving as instructed as soon as possible following surgery, to prevent blood clots from forming and to ease you into recovery. You will likely remain in the hospital for three days or longer after surgery. Your release depends on your physical condition, the extent of the surgery, and your progress in healing.

Cautions and Considerations

All of the complications and risks associated with breast surgery and with surgery in general are possible (see Question 19). In addition, if infection should develop and is not treated immediately you risk necrosis (pathologic death of one or more cells), or loss of the flap, and perhaps even the surrounding healthy tissue.

A pedicled TRAM is one of the most common and preferred methods of breast reconstruction where it is appropriate. It offers the most natural appearing breast, and one that feels natural to the touch. In some cases, you may regain what seems like normal sensations in your reconstructed breast. However, no reconstructed breast—including a pedicled TRAM—is an exact substitute for the breast that you lost. The initial shape and position of your breast may settle somewhat, and secondary procedures may be needed for final shaping of the breast.

Back to Life

Within two to four weeks following a pedicled TRAM reconstruction, you may be ready to get back to a moderate, daily routine. Exercise is an important part of your recovery, but it is important to follow the instructions you are given by your plastic surgeon or a physical therapist very closely. Too little exercise may hinder your recovery and too much may result in unnecessary injury. A side benefit to a pedicled TRAM procedure is that the patient will gain a modified **tummy tuck**, which is the removal of skin and fat from the abdomen and results in a slimmer profile.

A pedicled TRAM reconstruction has not been found to hinder monitoring breast health in any way, whether it is through breast self-exam or mammography. In fact, it has been found that if breast cancer should recur, it often does so near the incision sites and therefore may be more readily detected. Continuous follow-ups as recommended with your surgeon, oncologist, and plastic surgeon are your best defense to leading a healthy life and feeling whole.

60. What is a free flap reconstruction?

Unlike a pedicled TRAM or latissimus flap that remains tethered to its original blood supply, free flaps are flaps of skin and fat, and in some cases muscle, which are completely detached from the original site and reattached using microsurgical techniques to form a breast mound. The general types of free flaps used in breast reconstruction include:

- *Free TRAM (transverse rectus abdominus musculocutaeneous) flap*: taken from the abdomen like a pedi-

Tummy tuck
surgical procedure that removes skin and fat from the abdomen, resulting in a slimmer profile.

Free TRAM (transverse rectus abdominus musculocutaneous) flap
type of free flap breast reconstruction where a flap of skin, fat, and sometimes muscle are taken from the abdomen like a pedicled TRAM, but are completely detached from the abdomen; used to reform the breast.

cled TRAM, but completely detached from the abdomen

- **DIEP (deep inferior epigastric perforator) flap**: also taken from the abdomen, however, does not include the rectus muscle
- **GAP (gluteal artery perforator) flap**: taken from the gluteus or buttocks, using skin and fat from the superior gluteal (S-GAP) or inferior gluteal (I-GAP) regions
- **SIEA (superficial inferior epigastric artery)** perforator flap: taken from the abdomen, but avoids the rectus muscle

Some surgeons may also perform free flaps using tissue taken from the upper and midthigh. The use of flaps from the thigh is uncommon because they may leave conspicuous scars and are less reliable than other methods.

Good Candidates

Nearly every generally healthy woman is a good candidate for free flap reconstruction; the exception is women who are very thin. Among the advantages to free flaps is that they are appropriate in bilateral (both sides) cases of breast reconstruction and, depending upon the donor site, may cause little or no weakness to the muscles in the region where the flap was taken.

Women who have chronic illnesses that may impair healing, such as diabetes or connective tissue disorders such as lupus, may not be good candidates for any breast reconstruction with flap surgery. In addition, if you smoke, you are not a good candidate for reconstruction of any kind and will be advised to quit smoking before any reconstructive procedure and for many

---

DIEP (deep inferior epigastric perforator) flap

type of free flap breast reconstruction where a flap of skin and fat are taken from the abdomen, however, does not include the rectus muscle.

GAP (gluteal artery perforator) flap

type of free flap breast reconstruction where skin and fat are taken from the gluteus or buttocks, from the superior gluteal (S-GAP) or inferior gluteal (I-GAP) regions.

SIEA (superficial inferior epigastric artery) perforator flap

type of breast reconstruction where skin and fat are taken from the abdomen, avoiding the rectus muscle.

weeks following. To quit smoking for life is in the best interests of your health (see Question 22).

Surgery Experience

Like all flap procedures, a free flap is also performed under general anesthesia as an inpatient hospital procedure. The procedure will take several hours if performed at the time of mastectomy, or if delayed following mastectomy.

An incision at the flap donor site (the region where the flap is taken) will be made from which skin, fat, and blood vessels will be detached or harvested. In some cases, muscle may also be a component of the flap. The flap is completely separated from the donor site and positioned through the mastectomy incisions on the chest wall. Advanced microsurgical techniques are used to re-attach the blood vessels from the donor site to those at the chest wall. Internal sutures shape the breast and the incisions are then closed.

Following Surgery

You will awaken from surgery with a full breast mound in place. Thin, flexible tubes may be placed in your incisions to drain any excess fluid that collects. You will experience discomfort, swelling, and tenderness at the new breast site and the donor site.

It is important to begin moving as instructed as soon as possible following surgery, to prevent blood clots from forming and to ease you into recovery. You will remain in the hospital for two to five days or more. Your release depends on your physical condition, the extent of the surgery, and your progress in healing.

Cautions and Considerations

Free flap procedures are lengthy surgical processes. Depending on the flap donor site, a bilateral reconstruction may be recommended in two separate surgeries, one to reconstruct each breast, or performed on both breasts at the same time. All of the complications and risks associated with breast surgery and with surgery in general are possible (see Question #19). In addition, if infection should develop and is not treated immediately, you risk necrosis (pathologic loss of one or more cells), of loss the skin flap, and perhaps even surrounding healthy tissue.

Free flap procedures may result in some physical sensation in the breast; however, it will take some time to develop or for you to recognize. In addition, the initial shape and position of your breast may settle somewhat, and secondary procedures may be needed to refine breast appearance.

Back to Life

The recovery from a free flap procedure is variable, depending on a unilateral or bilateral reconstruction, the number of surgeries performed, and your overall health. You may be ready to get back to a moderate daily routine within two weeks following surgery. but you also may require a little more time. Exercise is an important part of your recovery. It is important to follow the instructions that you are given by your plastic surgeon or a physical therapist very closely. Too little exercise may hinder your recovery, and too much may result in unnecessary injury.

Because free flaps are composed of only natural tissue, they do not readily interfere with monitoring breast health or the presence or recurrence of breast cancer. Your breast health is best addressed by regular follow-up visits and screening with your surgeon, oncologist, and plastic surgeon.

61. How will my nipple and areola be reconstructed?

Nipple and areola reconstruction is the final phase of breast reconstruction. The nipple and areola are most often reconstructed in a secondary procedure that may be performed in your plastic surgeon's office or in an operating room. There are cases were the nipple is reconstructed at the time of initial breast reconstruction, although this is less common.

In order to create the projection of the nipple, small, localized skin flaps at the nipple site are elevated and sutured together. Incisions used to create the flaps will result in a scar that is hidden at the base of the nipple or in the region of the areola. In other cases, your plastic surgeon may take grafts of skin from the abdomen or inner thigh to reconstruct the areola. Here, the scars that result from attaching the grafts are concealed at the base of the nipple and outer border of the new areola.

Reconstruction of the areola (the darker pigmented skin surrounding the nipple) is achieved through grafting as noted above and/or specialized tattooing techniques. Your plastic surgeon will likely refer you to a medical tattoo specialist, or have a resource in his or her office to provide you this service.

62. What are my rights for coverage of breast reconstruction?

Most women do not know—and often are not told— that insurance companies are required by law to cover *any* procedures of breast reconstruction and ablative

surgery (partial or full mastectomy). This includes procedures determined by your plastic surgeon to achieve
symmetry between the breasts following lumpectomy,
mastectomy, or reconstruction. The enactment of this
law is directly a result of the patient advocacy efforts
led by the American Society of Plastic Surgeons that
not only mandated coverage for breast reconstruction,
but also for additional procedures on the opposite
breast necessary for achieving symmetry. Today, any
woman who undergoes mastectomy is entitled to coverage for reconstruction by her insurer. Pre-certification
may be required, and your surgeon's office will provide
the documentation necessary for coverage or assist you
in filing for insurance coverage.

The exact text of the 1998 Federal Breast Reconstruction Law and any updates to the law can be accessed
on the Web site, *www.plasticsurgery.org*, under "reconstructive procedures," "breast reconstruction," and then
"resources."

The American Society of Plastic Surgeons maintains a
state-by-state update of laws related to breast reconstruction on the Web site, *www.plasticsurgery.org*, under
"reconstructive procedures," "breast reconstruction,"
and then "resources."

63. Will my reconstructed breast match my other breast?

Part of the reconstruction consultation and your plastic
surgeon's expertise includes evaluating the best reconstruction techniques for your individual circumstances,
including the shape, size, and position of your opposite
breast. Symmetry is a factor; however, it remains possi-

ble that your reconstructed breast will not match your other breast. Breast reconstruction using an implant often results in a higher, firmer, more rounded breast compared to your natural breast. Breast reconstruction using flap surgery results in a softer, more natural breast than an implant, but still may never exactly match your natural breast.

Symmetry to your opposite breast should not be a concern or consideration to deter you from a recommended reconstruction procedure or from reconstruction in general. In your evaluation for reconstruction, your plastic surgeon will be able to tell you if surgery to the opposite breast would help you to achieve better symmetry. These procedures include:

- **Mastopexy** (breast lift) to raise and reshape a flat, sagging breast
- **Reduction mammaplasty** (breast reduction) to reduce the size of a large breast
- **Augmentation mammaplasty** (breast augmentation) to enhance the size of the breast by placing an implant

You may choose to have these secondary procedures performed at the time of reconstruction, or at a later date. No matter your choice, the same laws that require your insurer to cover breast reconstruction also require coverage of procedures prescribed to achieve symmetry.

64. What if I choose not to undergo breast reconstruction?

Breast reconstruction is entirely your choice. In many cases, the timing for reconstruction is your choice, too. Don't make your decision until you have had the

Mastopexy
a breast lift surgery to raise and reshape a flat, sagging breast.

Reduction mammaplasty
a breast reduction to reduce the size of a large breast.

Augmentation mammaplasty
a breast augmentation to enhance the size of the breast by surgically placing an implant in the breast.

opportunity to weigh all of your options, including the option not to have reconstruction.

There are alternatives to breast reconstruction; however, there is no alternative to surgical reconstruction of the breast that allows a woman to have a breast that is part of the body. An **external prosthesis** is a non-surgical alternative held in place by an undergarment. It is not part of a woman's body. This type of prosthesis may be uncomfortable and prevent a woman from wearing certain kinds of clothing. In addition, you may choose simply to live with the figure you have. That is entirely your choice. But know that in order to make a fully informed decision, you must be educated about all of your options. Take the time to consult with a plastic surgeon and consider breast reconstruction. It is your right, your personal self-image, and your satisfaction that can lead you to feel whole again.

According to a study reported by the American Cancer Society in November 2000, which was led by researchers at the University of Michigan, "Women who have breast reconstruction after a mastectomy report significant psychological and emotional benefits." Timing of breast reconstruction was reported to affect those benefits; however, the techniques used—with or without placement of a breast implant—did not appear to make much of a difference in a woman's level of satisfaction.

External prosthesis

a non-surgical alternative after breast surgery, that is a padded, artificial breast that is held in place by an undergarment.

PART SEVEN

Breast Reduction

What can be done to make my breasts smaller?

Why would I want to make my breasts smaller?

Do all women with large breasts experience pain?

More ...

65. *What can be done to make my breasts smaller?*

Breast reduction is surgery that removes fat and/or glandular tissue to reduce size and reshape a woman's breasts. While it is most often performed on women who have overly large, pendulous breasts—a condition called **macromastia**—some women choose breast reduction simply to bring better proportion to the female figure.

Don't mistake breast reduction as a procedure for women who are overweight. Breast size is primarily determined by heredity, but can be influenced by a woman's weight. While engaging in a healthy and active lifestyle may be difficult if you have overly large breasts, women who are significantly overweight may likely be advised to first achieve a healthy, stable weight, and then undergo breast reduction. The reason is simple: As weight fluctuates, so too will your breast size fluctuate. Having breast surgery when you are at a stable weight is likely to produce results that are stable as well.

In addition to the influences of weight on breast size, pregnancy and hormonal changes also may influence breast size. Some women develop larger breasts during pregnancy that remain large post-partum (after the baby is born), and this is as normal an occurrence as other women who lose breast volume post-partum. Some women experience hormonal changes in life that result in significant changes in breast size, and this may not be a normal occurrence. If you have had a sudden change in breast size without having changes in weight or a recent pregnancy, it is best to first have a complete health evaluation with your primary provider

Breast reduction

procedure to make large breasts smaller.

Macromastia

a condition characterized by overly large, pendulous breasts.

to ensure that breast size is not related to an illness or hormonal imbalance.

I grew up with friends who said they wished they had larger breasts. Well believe me, bigger is not always better. The stares and comments have always affected my confidence, and the physical restrictions to my life were not something I wanted to continue to accept. They say that sometimes small changes can make a big difference. Well, I don't think this was small change, and I know it made a big difference. Most importantly, it was right for me.

—Lauren

66. Why would I want to make my breasts smaller?

Only you can determine if you want to make your breasts smaller. This is a very important decision in your life, and requires research, consultation with a board-certified plastic surgeon, and a great deal of personal thought. Research indicates that women who do choose breast reduction are immensely satisfied by the experience, and that following breast reduction a woman's quality of life is greatly improved.

If you ever desired smaller breasts, or felt that your breast size has negatively influenced your self-esteem or quality of life, take the time to answer these statements with a simple "yes" or "no":

- I am self-conscious of my size breast size.
- My breast size impairs my ability to participate in certain physical activities.
- It is difficult for me to find clothing that fits or to wear the clothing styles that I want to wear.

- I avoid intimacy because of my breasts.
- I am embarrassed, or I have been ridiculed because of my breast size.
- My bra straps leave deep groves in my shoulders.
- I have sloping shoulders and/or a hunched-over posture.
- I experience frequent back, neck, shoulder, or arm pain.
- I experience breast pain.
- I have had rashes under my breastfold.
- My breasts are not symmetric (they are not equal in proportion, position, size, or shape).

If you answer "yes" to any of these questions, take a little more time to detail your answer or experience. Then you may wish to discuss your concerns with your personal physician first, but certainly take the time to consult with a board-certified plastic surgeon. Plastic surgeons are the only surgical specialists with training specific to changing the size, shape, and proportion of a woman's breasts, and this specifically includes breast reduction.

The American Society of Plastic Surgeons conducted a study funded by the Plastic Surgery Educational Foundation called BRAVO (breast reduction assessment and value outcomes) in 1999 to help measure the effectiveness and patient satisfaction of breast reduction surgery. The study specifically addressed women with macromastia, a D-cup or larger, who underwent breast reduction. Evidence showed that breast reduction patients experienced health-related, quality-of-life improvements following surgery, including a significant reduction of physical pain, and a boost in self-esteem and physical activity.

67. Do all women with large breasts experience pain?

Pain in the back, neck, shoulder, arms, or breasts is a common symptom of macromastia, but women don't always make the connection to these symptoms and their breast size. However, large pendulous breasts can cause stress on the back, neck, and shoulder muscles that keep a woman upright and support the weight of her breasts. For this reason, it is often advised that a woman with large breasts work actively to keep her back strong and healthy. But breast size can in fact hinder a woman's ability to engage in many forms of exercise. In addition, the strain on bra straps can cut into the shoulders, causing deep grooves and sometimes even bruising. Over time, this can affect the thoracic outlet, a nerve center running through the neck and shoulder. Thoracic outlet syndrome commonly presents as numbness and tingling in the fingers, weakness in the arms, and, literally, a pain in the neck.

There is no standard for what size breast causes pain of any kind or severity, just as there is no standard for the size, shape, and physical condition of all women. A very small-framed woman may experience pain from a much smaller breast size than a woman with a larger frame, broader shoulders, or stronger stance. Equally, a very large-framed woman with a weak back or other over-riding conditions such as arthritis or scoliosis may suffer immense pain from her breasts, where a healthy woman of similar size may have few, if any, symptoms of pain.

If you have overly large breasts, or a breast size that you feel self-conscious about, breast reduction is equally as appropriate in your case as in the case of a woman who experiences significant pain. However, while breast reduction is considered a reconstructive procedure—one to restore a more normal appearance and to improve a physical condition and a woman's health and quality of life—in those cases where it is simply your desire to reduce breast size, the procedure may be considered aesthetic, simply to enhance your goals for your appearance.

I didn't have physical pain all the time, but I did always experience pain. I wouldn't wear a bathing suit much less a sweater, and felt people were always looking at my breasts, not me. I couldn't look a man in the eye and that was more difficult to take than the physical pain.

—Lauren

68. What can I expect during breast reduction?

Breast reduction is surgery that removes excess fat, skin, and glandular tissue to reduce breast size and reshape overly large breasts. The weight of overly large breasts can cause skin to become severely stretched, and result in breasts that are pendulous or saggy. In addition, overly large breasts often lack firmness and therefore not only sag, but also are flattened on the top, with all the weight of the breast hanging like a baseball in a sock. By reducing breast size, tightening breast tissue, and removing excess skin, breast reduction can reduce, reshape, and reposition the breasts to a more normal size, more rounded shape, and natural, outward projection. Achieving a reduced size and more normal breast shape most often requires repositioning the nipple and areola during breast reduction. In some cases your plastic surgeon may recommend, or you may choose, to have an enlarged areola reduced.

Good Candidates

Breast reduction candidates are generally women whose physical development has matured, generally after the age of 16 years. However, breast development, including changes in breast size, can occur throughout life. Therefore, if you undergo breast reduction at an early age, it may likely be that your breasts will continue to grow or change, and you may need or desire additional reduction later in life.

In addition, good candidates for breast reduction are generally healthy women with no diseases that may impair healing such as diabetes, autoimmune diseases, or connective tissue disorders. Women who smoke, use any tobacco products, or consume large amounts of alcohol are not good candidates for breast reduction, and will be advised to stop for several weeks or months prior to surgery. If you fail to stop smoking and choose to undergo breast reduction, then you are putting yourself at a serious increased risk of complication and severely impairing your ability to heal properly (see Question 22). It is your responsibility to follow the instructions you are given to the letter, and to advise your plastic surgeon if you have not followed these instructions. Your outcomes depend on your total compliance with all of the instructions you are given.

Surgery Experience

Breast reduction is almost always performed under general anesthesia and may be performed on an outpatient basis, or you may be advised to remain in the hospital or a special overnight care facility for a day or two following surgery.

Breast Reduction

Surgery requires incisions for your plastic surgeon to excise (remove) excess breast fat, skin, and glandular tissue. These incisions will leave visible scars on the breast, however, the scars are concealed by most bras and swimsuit tops. In general, the incision patterns include:

- A keyhole pattern encircling the nipple and areola, extending downward and under the breast to just at the breast crease, and extending horizontally just about the level of the breast crease. This results in a scar pattern that looks like an anchor. It encircles the perimeter of the areola (where a well-healed scar is highly unnoticeable), in a straight line down to the breast crease, and horizontally in a slightly curved line just at the breast crease.

- A racquet shaped pattern, which is similar to the keyhole pattern, eliminates most or all of the horizontal incision just above the breast crease. The resulting scar encircles the areola and forms a straight line from the base of the areola to the base of the breast. Sometimes a small incision may be used at the base of the breast to reduce excess tissue in this region.

- A concentric or donut shaped pattern that encircles the areola and extends in a perimeter just beyond the areola. This pattern leaves no visible scarring on the breast surface; however, in cases where breasts are pendulous, or slope downward quite a bit, this technique may not produce an optimal final shape. Also, the concentric pattern is a bit of a misnomer as the actual donut removed may be somewhat wider or narrower on either the top or bottom of the areola, depending on your current breast shape and the degree of correction necessary to achieve a good outcome.

- A horizontal incision just about the level of the breast crease only. This technique is much less commonly practiced.

An incision around the areola allows the nipple and areola to remain attached to the underlying nerves, vessels, and tissue in what is considered a local flap. This is an area of tissue that remains attached to its original blood supply and is merely repositioned to a new location upward. The fat and glands that are not part of the flap are carefully excised (removed) to reduce breast volume, and underlying tissues are shaped with internal sutures.

In cases where the skin is deeply sagging, such as in very large breasts, the nipple and areola may need to be removed completely and grafted to a more natural position. This is not at all common (with the exception of very large, pendulous breasts) and should be avoided, if possible. A nipple that is grafted will not regain sensation and there is also the risk of losing the nipple entirely if the graft does not heal.

In some cases, your plastic surgeon may include the use of liposuction to remove excess fat in and around the breast. This is generally an adjunct procedure and is rarely used as the sole method to achieve breast reduction (Figure 4).

Following Surgery

When you awaken from breast reduction, you may have small, thin drainage tubes coming from each breast, as determined by your surgeon. Your breasts will likely be wrapped in a compression or support bra, and

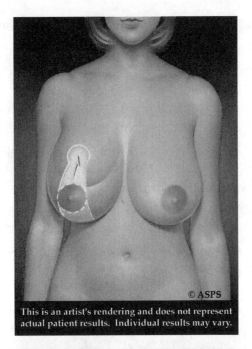

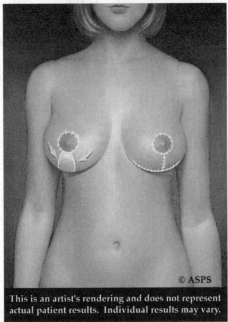

Figure 4 **Breast Reduction (reduction mammaplasty). Courtesy of the American Society of Plastic Surgeons®. All rights reserved. Learn more at *www.plasticsurgery.org*.**

you will experience discomfort localized to the breast region. This can easily be controlled with medication.

In addition, you will be instructed to begin moving about and walking as soon as possible to reduce the risk of blood clot formation. Despite any discomfort and bandages or special garments, you will immediately notice that your breasts are lighter and smaller.

Cautions and Considerations

All of the cautions and considerations associated with any type of surgery, and with breast surgery in general, are possible with breast reduction (see Question 19). In addition, it is possible that following surgery your breasts may not be completely symmetric. Minor asymmetry between the breasts is perfectly normal for most women and is often only detectable to you. However, significant asymmetry in breast size or shape is possible and may require additional surgery to correct.

In addition, breast tissue is very soft and susceptible to healing with scars that can become raised, red, wide, or stressed. It is very important to follow all of the wound care instructions you are given, and instructions for wearing your support bra or compression. In the first few weeks following surgery, it is likely you will be directed to wear some form of breast support around the clock.

You should also be advised that breast reduction can variably influence your future ability to breast-feed. This is most often the case where breast size is mostly attributed to excess mammary glands and when reduction requires removing some of the mammary glands. However, it is not fully predictable whether a woman will be able to breast-feed following breast reduction.

Therefore, if you are planning future pregnancies, be advised that your ability to breast-feed may be impaired. Although breast reduction techniques that do not graft the nipple and areola usually result in a normal sensation of the nipple, changes in sensation can occur with some women noting an increase, decrease, or total loss of sensation.

Back to Life

While it may take one to two weeks before you are ready to get back to a normal daily routine, any physical pain or discomfort caused by your overly large breast will likely improve rapidly following your breast reduction. You will definitely stand taller and have an improved posture and confidence. You may want to get into a new fitness routine and enjoy the activities that were very uncomfortable or difficult prior to your breast reduction. However, don't engage in any physical activity until your plastic surgeon gives you clearance to do so. Your newly reduced breasts will need time to heal and settle into their new position. To engage in strenuous physical activity, and to push, pull, lift, or swing your arms with any force may injure delicate breast tissue as it heals.

Even though your breast shape will settle a bit, you can begin shopping for new fashions and new bras as soon as you feel ready. Don't wear underwire bras until you are advised by your physician. Remember that your new, better-proportioned figure is only enhanced by maintaining a stable weight and by good, stable support of your breasts, particularly during your fitness routine.

According to the American Society of Plastic Surgeons, in 2004, breast reduction was the fifth most common reconstructive plastic surgery procedure performed, with just over 105,592 procedures in the United States. This was a steady increase of 10,000 or more procedures over the preceding three years. The American Society for Aesthetic Plastic Surgery reported 125,600 procedures in that same year; the discrepancy is likely due to the fact that breast reduction was looked upon as a whole by ASAPS, not only as a reconstructive procedure.

69. Is there an alternative to surgical breast reduction?

In some cases, liposuction alone can reduce excess fat in the breast, but it won't reshape a breast that has become pendulous, nor will it improve the position of the nipple and areola, or improve the shape and size of an enlarged areola. Liposuction alone is more often appropriate in limited cases of reduction, that is, those cases that are more for aesthetic reasons (stemming from a desire to improve your appearance) than for reduction to improve your physical condition and quality of life.

There really is no other means to reduce breast size than surgical reduction. Creams can only firm the texture or feel of the skin surface. They cannot tighten your breasts or melt, dissolve, or change the composition or amount of breast tissue. Weight loss can reduce breast size by reducing weight overall, but this may not necessarily affect the amount of excess glandular breast tissue you have. Physical exercises may strengthen and tighten the underlying pectoral muscles, or improve the strength and condition of your back and shoulders, but they will do nothing to reduce breast size or the excess weight of your breasts and resulting pressure on your neck, shoulders, and back. Minimizing bras may or may not be helpful, but may even contribute to your symptoms. Only surgical breast reduction can improve breast size and improve your physical symptoms and quality of life.

70. What are my rights regarding breast reduction coverage?

Unfortunately, at present there is no legislation that affords a woman the right to insurance coverage for breast reduction in certain cases, nor are there insurance industry standards. Most commonly, the standards for reimbursement or insurance coverage of breast reduction are defined by the insurer and are based on the volume of breast tissue to be removed and other criteria (such as height, weight, previous medical treatment for pain, etc.). Some insurers may deny coverage altogether.

Debate and lobbying for a uniform standard among insurers for coverage of breast reduction has been an ongoing effort of the American Society of Plastic Surgeons. However, the most appropriate standard would have to take into account the proportion of breast size to a woman's body. Many insurers base their decisions for breast reduction coverage on the amount of tissue removed from each breast. The amount is arbitrary and does not take into consideration that smaller women may suffer immense physical symptoms from breasts that are not nearly as large as a more moderate woman. Standards based on the volume of reduction also don't take into consideration the physical symptoms a woman is experiencing.

The best approach you can take toward obtaining coverage for your breast reduction is to first:

- Read your health insurance policy for language specific to breast surgery or breast reduction, and to determine your policy limitations or pre-certification requirements.
- Discuss, document, and have a full evaluation of the physical symptoms you experience due to your breast size with your primary care physician, and with an orthopedic or back specialist, if necessary. Confer with these health care providers on their recommendation for breast reduction to improve your condition, and ask them to document their recommendations with your health insurance company.
- Consult with a board-certified plastic surgeon and have that plastic surgeon's office provide your insurer with all of the documentation and information necessary to pre-certify your breast reduction.

If a breast reduction is clearly in the best interests of improving the physical symptoms you experience as a result of your overly large breasts, no insurer should deny you coverage. Unfortunately, sometimes they do. Be persistent.

If your breast reduction is something you seek personally to improve your body image, you need to bear the cost of that surgery. While the difference between these cases should be very clear to you, they are often not judged clearly by insurers. Therefore, be patient with the documentation your insurer requires, and be persistent about your right to improve your quality of life and your health.

While insurance coverage for breast reduction is variable, there are women who, despite the lack or denial of coverage, proceed with the procedure and pay for it themselves. This is entirely your choice. You need to consider the value the procedure has to your overall health and quality of life.

71. How can breast reduction improve my life?

Greater mobility and a likely reduction of the pain experiences from having overly large breasts are the greatest benefits to your life. As a result, you can benefit from the ability to participate in and enjoy many more physical and fitness activities, which can only enhance your health even further.

You will also find yourself less self-conscious of your body image, and likely will be much more confident of yourself. You won't feel that others are staring at your breast size and you will enjoy the freedom to wear anything you wish.

As part of the BRAVO breast reduction assessment study conducted by the American Society of Plastic Surgeons, cases studies were conducted in which women described their experiences following breast reduction. These case studies represent an unbiased and direct perspective on quality-of-life improvements following breast reduction surgery. These case studies can be accessed through the Web site, *www.plasticsurgery.org,* under "reconstructive procedures," "breast reduction," and "BRAVO."

72. Can breast reduction affect my breast health?

In addition to relieving the physical symptoms resulting from large breasts as well as boosting your self image and self-esteem, breast reduction may have additional, positive affects on your health.

In a May 2004 study published by the *Plastic and Reconstructive Surgery Journal*, women who suffered from macromastia and who were without underlying factors that elevated their risk of developing breast cancer actually experienced a reduction in the risk of developing breast cancer overall, following breast reduction surgery. This was the first study of its kind. While these preliminary results are encouraging and certainly support that breast reduction can improve a woman's health, it is not yet conclusive to say that breast reduction does, in fact, reduce a woman's chances of developing breast cancer. Future research is needed to fully validate these outcomes. In addition, it has been reported that women who have had breast reduction are more confident in their monthly breast self-exams; as there is less tissue to evaluate, the changes in the breasts can be more readily recognized.

PART EIGHT

Breast Augmentation

How can my breasts be enlarged?

Why would I want larger breasts?

What are my options for breast augmentation?

More ...

73. How can my breasts be enlarged?

The most common way to permanently enlarge the size of your breasts is through the surgical placement of a breast implant, called breast augmentation, or **augmentation mammaplasty**.

Augmentation mammaplasty

surgery to enhance breast size through the placement of a breast implant.

There are alternatives to enhance the appearance of breast size. A woman can wear padded bras or place inserts or padding into her bra. There are push-up, pump-up, and Wonder bras® marketed to make breasts look larger. A number of pill type supplements, creams, devices, and exercises have been purported to increase breast size. None of these are permanent *and* are a part of your own body. None of the marketed devices and herbal supplements to enhance breast size has been proven to achieve permanent breast enhancement. These are not subject to U.S. Food and Drug Administration (FDA) approval or marketing regulations, and therefore their claims are unproven in unbiased clinical studies. Additionally, there are rare circumstances where a patient's own body tissue may be used for augmentation, but this is very uncommon. Breast implants are the primary choice to increase breast size.

Therefore, if you wish to enlarge your breast size permanently, and in a fashion that is part of your own body, the only means to do so is through surgical insertion of breast implants.

Breast augmentation is the most commonly performed aesthetic plastic surgery procedure for women in the United States, as reported by the American Society for Aesthetic Plastic Surgery. Over 332,000 procedures were performed in 2004, which was a 230% increase since 1997.

74. Why would I want larger breasts?

Only you can answer the question of why you want larger breasts. The most common reasons women desire breast augmentation are:

* Breast size is genetically small
* Breast size has diminished following pregnancy and/or nursing
* Breast size is small in proportion to the structure and size of the body, overall
* To enhance what is an otherwise normal breast size
* To correct a minor asymmetry (difference in size) of the breasts

The more important questions you should ask of yourself are:

* What do I expect from a breast augmentation?
* What is my motivation for wanting a breast augmentation?
* Is my decision my own?
* Am I willing to accept that maintaining my breast appearance and health is a lifetime commitment, even though breast implants are not lifetime devices?

If you expect that breast augmentation will do anything more than give you the personal confidence and satisfaction in your own body that you want, reconsider your expectations. Breast augmentation cannot make a failing relationship better, nor can it win you the job or the situation in life you want. These things can only occur as the result of your own motivation and behaviors, not larger breasts.

Your motivation for wanting larger breasts, much like your expectations, should be for your own personal satisfaction, and not that of anyone else. Your decision to have breast implants should be yours alone. Don't do it because your partner or significant other likes large-breasted women, or because you feel social pressure to achieve a bigger bra size. Most importantly, you need to accept that having breast augmentation is a lifetime commitment.

- It requires specialized mammography for more accurate screening of breast health.
- It requires periodic visits to your plastic surgeon to evaluate the condition of your implants and your breasts.
- As your body changes over time, the appearance of your breasts may change, and your implants may need to be replaced with a modified style or placement to maintain a natural appearance.
- Should implants rupture, leak, or deflate, the implants must be replaced or you may face having disfigured breasts.
- If capsular contracture (a constricting scar tissue that squeezes the implant and produces an unnatural appearance and can be painful) develops, it may require surgery to correct and that implants be replaced.

The U.S. FDA defines that breast implants are not lifetime devices and, therefore, you need to accept that it is likely, at some point in life, you will either desire or need to have your implants replaced.

In 2004, the American Society of Plastic Surgeons (ASPS) reported that 35,208 breast implants for augmentation purposes only were removed, and that 81%

of those were replaced. The most common reasons for implant removal were (1) a change in breast size and (2) implant rupture or leakage.

75. What are my options for breast augmentation?

Your options for breast augmentation are basically: the type of implant and filler; the size of the implant; placement of incisions; and the placement of the breast implant.

To understand all of the options available for you in breast implants, and all that is associated with breast implants, read Part 4: Breast Implants (Questions 26–39). In general, with an augmentation your choices are:

- Saline-filled or silicone implants
- The size of the implant necessary to achieve your desired final breast size
- The shape of the implant
- The type of implant shell: smooth or textured
- If saline, whether the implant is pre-filled or filled at the time of placement
- Incision placement:
  - Just in or above the natural crease of the lower breast
  - In the axilla (underarm area)
  - Along the lower perimeter of the areola (the dark skin surrounding the nipple)
- Placement of the implant:
  - Sub-mammary (also called sub-glandular) placement: below the breast tissue and on top of the pectoral muscles

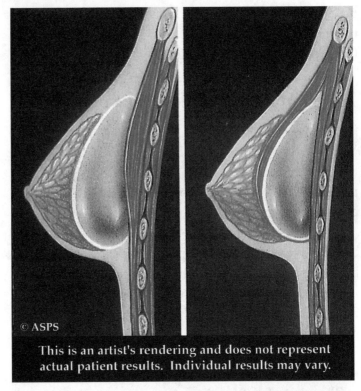

This is an artist's rendering and does not represent actual patient results. Individual results may vary.

Figure 5   Breast Augmentation. (a) subglandular; (b) submuscular. Courtesy of the American Society of Plastic Surgeons®. All rights reserved. Learn more at *www.plasticsurgery.org*.

- Submuscular (also called sub-pectoral) placement: under the pectoral muscles (Figure 5)

You might have an idea of what you wish your final breast size to be. Trying on various implant sizes in your bra may be helpful, or trying on various bra sizes and padding them is helpful, too. But you and your plastic surgeon together should consider a few things before making a decision: your body frame and proportion, the stability of your weight, the current amount of your natural breast tissue, and skin elasticity. You must have ample breast tissue to cover the implant even if the implant will be placed under the muscle, or the results may include rippling, stretch marks, an unnatural appearance, extrusion of the implant (it becomes visible on the surface), or an increased risk of capsular contracture. If your weight fluctuates significantly, so too, can your breast size and shape fluctuate.

Incision placement often depends on the type of implant placed, where it is placed, and the techniques used.

- Most common is a 2–3 inch incision depending on implant size, just a hairline above the natural breast crease.
- Implants placed through a 1.5-inch incision or smaller in the axilla, and may be placed through the use of an **endoscope** (a hollow surgical tube) and then filled with saline once positioned.
- Implants placed along the bottom edge of the areola. There is an alternative method called **TUBA (transumbilical breast augmentation)** that uses an endoscope placed through an incision in the navel to place and fill saline breast implants. This is highly controversial and should not be considered a routine incision site for the placement of breast implants (Figure 6).

Sub-mammary placement of the implant (below the breast tissue) generally has a somewhat shorter recovery. During upper body activity and exercise, sub-mammary placed implants can be somewhat obvious. Placement of the implant under the pectoral muscle has a somewhat longer recovery, and a more naturally sloped appearance. **Sub-muscular** implants may also make post-augmentation mammography easier to interpret.

Breast Augmentation

Endoscope

a type of microsurgical instrument that is basically a hollow tube. An implant can be placed in the breast and then filled using this tool.

TUBA (trans umbilical breast augmentation)

a type of breast augmentation technique that uses an endoscope placed through an incision in the navel, to place and fill saline breast implants. This is highly controversial and should not be considered a routine incision site for the placement of breast implants.

Sub-mammary

below the breast tissue; some implants are placed in that location.

Sub-muscular

below the muscle; some implants are placed under the pectoral muscle.

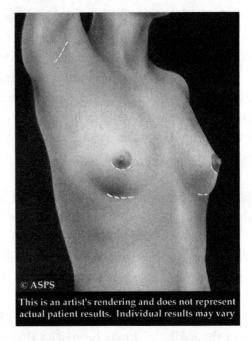

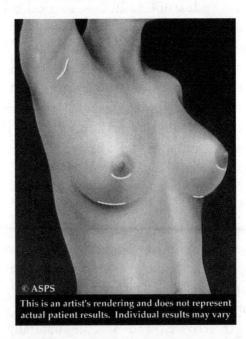

Figure 6   Breast Augmentation. Courtesy of the American Society of Plastic Surgeons®. All rights reserved. Learn more at *www.plasticsurgery.org*.

The choices you have are not yours alone to decide. This is a job for you and your plastic surgeon to discuss, and then to decide on together. You must have confidence in your plastic surgeon, the choices you have made, and in your overall decision before you proceed with breast augmentation.

Questions 36 and 37 discuss capsular contracture and risks comprehensively. Read these questions and the entire section on breast implants carefully.

76. What can I expect during breast augmentation?

Before you actually have surgery, you can expect to feel some anxiety, some excitement, and some stress. But the most important thing to do is be confident in your decision, follow all of your plastic surgeon's instructions, and get ready to toss away those padded bras!

Women who undergo breast augmentation by credentialed, skilled, experienced plastic surgeons report very high satisfaction, not only in appearance, but also in the way their breasts feel. Much of the key to your success in breast augmentation, as with any plastic surgery procedure, is to consult with a qualified, board-certified plastic surgeon. He or she should have experience in breast augmentation and other breast procedures. In addition, the surgeon you choose should listen carefully to your goals for surgery, that is, the physical change you want to achieve and your personal expectations for enhancing breast size (see Questions 7–11).

Good Candidates

Women of any age who are in good physical and emotional health are good candidates for breast augmentation. It should not, however, be performed in patients younger than 18 years unless severe asymmetry exists. If the breasts are severely **ptotic** (sagging), augmentation should not be performed without some form of mastopexy (breast lift); otherwise, your outcome may actually worsen the appearance of your breasts, rather than achieving naturally full and rounded breasts. If you are age 30 years or older, a baseline mammogram prior to augmentation is a good idea and may be required by your plastic surgeon. Smokers should refrain from smoking for several weeks or months before surgery and during recovery (see Question 22).

Ptosis

sagging, drooping, or falling tissues or organs.

Surgery Experience

Breast augmentation is most commonly an outpatient procedure performed either under general anesthesia or local anesthesia with sedation, in an office-based, freestanding, ambulatory, or hospital-based surgical facility. An overnight hospital stay may be recommended in some cases.

Your surgeon will make an incision based on your discussions and consent, and will create a pocket in which to place the implant. The implant will be placed, filled if it was not pre-filled, and the incisions will be closed.

Following Surgery

When you awaken from surgery, you will be stiff and sore. Tissues will be stretching to accommodate the breast implant and the swelling that occurs from the surgery itself. Most discomfort may be controlled with oral medications. Placement of a pain pump, which is a device that delivers medication directly to the surgical site, is very helpful to control discomfort during the first three days after surgery. In some cases, small, thin tubes may be placed at the incision sites to drain any excess fluid that might accumulate. You will be wearing a support bra, elastic bandage, or chest band for the first week or more following surgery, as recommended by your surgeon.

If you have had sub-mammary placement, you will be back to your daily routine in just a few days; add a few more days if the implant was placed sub-muscularly. You'll want to refrain from heavy exercise, twisting, pushing, pulling, or lifting until your plastic surgeon advises that you may ease into these activities. Proper wound care and subsequent breast massage as instructed by your plastic surgeon can help to avoid capsular contracture and unsightly scars. Wearing your support bra as directed is imperative to proper healing. Even when your surgeon allows you to discontinue wearing a support bra, you may find that wearing light support, like a shelf bra or camisole, to be comfortable for sleeping.

Cautions and Considerations

The risks and complications of breast augmentation include hematoma or blood pooling beneath the skin, breast tenderness, and heightened or lack of nipple sensation. There is a slight chance you may have unexpected milk production following insertion of implants. This may stop on its own or require medication. There is also the possibility of poorly healed or wide scars. Capsular contracture may develop (see Questions 36 and 37 for more on all the risks of breast implants). Implants can be displaced, leak, or rupture. If they become infected, they very likely will need to be removed. There are also the risks associated with anesthesia.

Once healing is completed, an annual examination with your plastic surgeon to assess the condition of your implants and your breasts is also important. You should also have an annual exam with your primary physician or gynecologist to check for breast changes and masses.

Back to Life

The results of breast augmentation are visible immediately, although you will be somewhat swollen and your implants will appear higher than you might wish your final outcome to be. It may take six to eight weeks or more before implants settle to a final position. By this time, you will be shopping for new sweaters, swimsuits, and bras. Breast augmentation generally should not interfere with a woman's ability to breast-feed, nor should it significantly alter the sensations in a woman's nipples. However, any surgery of the breast may result in these conditions.

Breast augmentation with implants has the advantage of slowing the natural aging or sagging process of the breasts in some women. However, where implant size is excessive, sagging and aging of the breasts may actually be exaggerated. Some women find they need not wear a bra, and find new freedom and satisfaction in the way clothing fits and in new clothing options to enhance their figures.

77. Is breast augmentation covered by insurance?

Breast augmentation is an aesthetic procedure. The only consideration for insurance coverage is to achieve symmetry in severely disproportionate breasts, or when the opposite breast has been reconstructed after surgery to remove all or a portion of the breast (mastectomy).

78. How can breast augmentation look or feel more natural?

Don't expect implants of any kind to feel totally natural. What you need to determine is whether the slight difference in the feeling of your breasts is a fair trade-off to achieving the size you want. You also need to decide if a few extra days of recovery are worth a much more natural result.

The best means to achieve the most natural results is through careful evaluation of all the appropriate options defined by your plastic surgeon. In general this means:

- Breast implants that are not overly large for the amount of natural breast tissue, and your body frame and proportion
- Breast implants in an appropriate shape to achieve your goals for final fullness and shape as well as projection or contour
- Sub-muscular placement of breast implants

Everyone is an individual, and all of your own physical characteristics and personal goals will help to determine the most natural outcomes for your breast augmentation.

While most agree that silicone implants feel more like natural breast tissue, to some women, the choice of a somewhat firmer breast with saline implants can be equally satisfying. Don't let anyone convince you that over- or underfilling saline implants can result in a more natural look. Implants are manufactured to defined specifications and approved by the U.S. FDA based on these specifications. Given all the options available, there is no need to deviate from appropriate practices.

79. Can breast augmentation improve sagging breasts, too?

Placement of implants alone may somewhat alter breast shape and improve firmness; however, low breast or nipple position can only be corrected through breast lift. This means that your breasts are more sloped than flat or they are slightly less perky than you would hope them to be. So, the answer to this question is a conditional "yes." It is conditional upon the degree of sagging, the cause of the sagging, and likely the progression over time as well as the degree of enhancement in breast size you desire. A naturally, slightly sloped breast can be enhanced in size, shape, and projection by the placement of breast implants.

If your sagging is the result of skin that has stretched due to fluctuations in breast size over time, or that your breasts are flat and sagging with nipples pointed downward, your plastic surgeon will likely recommend a breast lift in addition to the placement of implants to reduce skin and re-shape the breast in a more natural position. Part of your natural and successful outcomes in breast augmentation include placement of the implant in a pocket beneath the breast tissue or **pectoral muscle**. If the breast is sagging, an implant beneath the breast tissue will sag, too. An implant behind the pectoral muscle will look terribly unnatural; the implant would be positioned high on the chest wall, with sagging breast tissue and the nipple hanging below.

Your best option is a thorough consultation and examination by a board-certified plastic surgeon who is experienced in both breast augmentation and breast lift (see Questions 7–11).

For more information specifically on breast lift, read on to Part 9: Breast Lift.

Pectoral muscle
a type of muscle located in the chest.

Breast Augmentation

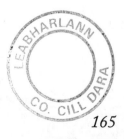

165

PART NINE

Breast Lift and Other Procedures

What can be done to improve sagging or flat breasts?

What can I expect after a breast lift?

Will a breast lift make my breasts smaller?

More . . .

80. What can be done to improve sagging or flat breasts?

Both the condition of breast skin, and the coinciding shape and position of the underlying tissue can result in breasts that sag and have a flattened shape. These conditions can be caused by heredity and aging. Sagging of the breast also can be the result of a reduction in breast volume, either from weight loss or changes of the breast associated with pregnancy and breast-feeding. In any case, poor elasticity of skin that has significantly stretched is a significant factor.

In higher degrees of ptosis, the nipple and areola of the breast hang lower than the breast crease, and the upper portion of the breast is flattened. Many women who experience severe ptosis must wear a support bra at all times to keep the breasts in a more normal position. In many cases, these women avoid swimsuits, certain fashions, and even intimacy because of the appearance of their breasts. Exercise can firm the underlying pectoral muscles of the breast, but do nothing to change the shape and position of mammary tissue and fat. Creams and massage can somewhat improve the surface of skin that has lost elasticity, but can do nothing to reduce severely stretched skin. In fact, there is no alternative to surgical breast lift. Only breast lift, also called mastopexy, has been proven to improve, raise, or restore breast shape.

Breast lift changes the breast to a more youthful shape and position. It repositions the nipple to a higher location, with a more natural point of projection. It can also reduce the size of the areola (the darker skin surrounding the nipple). In general, breast lift reshapes and uplifts the breasts and areolas, resulting in a more youthful and "perky" appearance. They have a naturally appearing, more rounded shape, outward projection, and neutral position. Following breast lift, a woman can feel confident and comfortable in any style of clothing or swimsuit, and with the appearance of her figure.

Breast lift is the least common of breast procedures. The American Society of Plastic Surgeons reported nearly 67,000 procedures performed in 2003.

81. What can I expect after a breast lift?

Breast lift restores firmness, reshapes the breast, and raises the breast and nipple to a higher, more natural position. It is surgery, and requires incisions made on the breast for your plastic surgeon to reshape the deep tissues of the breast and to reduce excess skin of the breast and areola. In general, they include one or a combination of all of the following incisions:

• Around the areola
• Extending vertically downward from the areola to the breast crease
• Horizontally in or just above the breast crease

Your incision pattern will be based on the amount of correction that will achieve your goals, the quality of your skin tone and amount of skin that must be reduced, the size of the areola, and the location of the nipple. If a reduction in the size of your areola is necessary, then you will require an incision around the perimeter of the areola. Not all incision patterns are appropriate in all cases. Therefore, a consultation and examination by a plastic surgeon with experience in breast lift procedures, and the variety of techniques and incision patterns of breast lift, is essential to determine what is right for you (Figure 7).

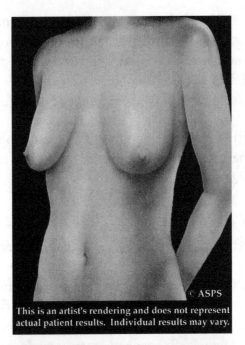

This is an artist's rendering and does not represent actual patient results. Individual results may vary.

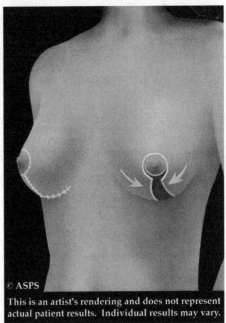

This is an artist's rendering and does not represent actual patient results. Individual results may vary.

Figure 7   Breast Lift (mastopexy). Courtesy of the American Society of Plastic Surgeons®. All rights reserved. Learn more at *www.plasticsurgery.org*.

Good Candidates

Any woman who desires to improve the shape and position of her breasts, who is in general good health, and who has realistic expectations for the outcomes of surgery, is a good candidate for breast lift. Women who may have future pregnancies might consider postponing a breast lift. Breast lift may not affect breast-feeding; however, the results of your surgery can be significantly diminished by the changes in the breasts that occur during pregnancy and breast-feeding.

Smoking can significantly affect your ability to heal, and any patient who smokes should stop smoking for several weeks before surgery and during recovery (see Question 22). Women considering breast lift need to understand that the improvement of breast shape and position is accompanied by permanent scarring on the breast. Additionally, breast lift does not reverse the effects of aging because less elastic skin and gravity on the breast and additional sagging (to some degree) are inevitable after surgery.

Surgery Experience

Breast lift most likely will be performed with general anesthesia, or local anesthesia with sedation. The procedure will be performed in an office-based, freestanding, ambulatory- or hospital-based surgical facility and is routinely done on an outpatient basis.

Through the incision pattern your surgeon defines appropriate for you, the underlying breast tissue will be fashioned to a more uplifted and rounded position and shape. Deep sutures may be used to hold the breast tissue in place. If necessary, the size of the areola is reduced in circumference. Excess breast skin is removed and the nipple is raised to a higher position. The skin is brought together and incisions closed to achieve your new breast shape and position.

You may awaken from surgery wearing a support bra or elastic bandage that you will continue to wear as recommended by your plastic surgeon. Small tubes may be placed at the incision sites to allow any excess fluid accumulation to drain; these will likely be in place for a few days. You will be sore and experience discomfort at the incision sites following surgery. However, this discomfort can easily be controlled with medication.

Following Surgery

You may resume light normal activity as soon as you feel ready, and should be walking on the day of surgery. But you will want to avoid lifting anything heavy, or making any jerking or pulling motions for the first few days following surgery. If you have non-absorbable sutures, they will be removed in a week or two following surgery. You may be given silicone tapes or gel to apply to your scars to reduce the formation of raised, red, firm, or other undesirable scars. You will continue wearing the support bra around the clock for several weeks, or as directed by your surgeon. You should avoid wearing underwire bras until permitted to do so by your plastic surgeon.

Cautions and Considerations

The results of breast lift surgery are visible immediately, although breast shape will continue to settle for several months. Final results, including the softening and fading of scars, may take as much as one to two years. Scars will always be visible, but they are usually hidden under most swimsuits and bras. The risks of breast lift include the development of thick or wide scars. Follow all instructions for wound cleansing, massage of scars, and the use of tapes or topical ointments. This can improve the appearance of scars and lessen the chance of forming raised or firm scars. Following all instructions for wearing support garments is essential to your breasts healing properly. Some women wear a support camisole when sleeping. If that is comfortable for you, it can only enhance and help to maintain the results of your breast lift.

An additional risk of breast lift surgery is blood pooling beneath the skin (hematoma) that may need to be drained, if possible. A loss of nipple sensation or temporary sensitivity is possible. There is also the risk of infection, but this is rare. As with any surgical procedure, there are risks associated with anesthesia.

Breast lift should not interfere with your ability to breast-feed, and will rarely alter normal breast sensations. Breast lift surgery is not completely permanent. Over time as the result of natural aging, breasts may sag or lose elasticity. You can help to maintain your results by maintaining a stable weight.

Back to Life

Women who undergo breast lift find new confidence not only in their appearance when clothed, but also without clothing, so long as they accept the visible scars that will remain on their breasts. Following breast lift, fashion choices and confidence are greatly increased. Any visible scars on the breast are easily concealed by most swimsuits and clothing. More youthful and shapely breast appearance can be very fulfilling and appealing from the shape of the figure overall to personal confidence in appearance.

82. Will a breast lift make my breasts smaller?

Breast lift does not normally change the volume of breasts, only breast shape and position. Following breast lift, you may find that you are wearing a somewhat smaller bra size, but this is not likely the result of a reduction, but rather your now firmer and rounder breast shape.

However, in some cases a very small reduction of breast volume may be performed on one or both breasts to achieve symmetry and to achieve good outcomes. Discuss this thoroughly with your plastic surgery. If your resulting breast size is as important to you as shape and position, then your discussion may include reduction of large breasts or the addition of an implant to enhance smaller breast size.

83. Why are breast implants sometimes placed with a breast lift?

A breast implant may be placed during a breast lift for several reasons:

- If you desire an enlargement along with your breast lift
- If the amount of breast tissue removed to achieve your uplift will result in a significant size reduction
- To result in an naturally firmer breast, overall

To determine if breast implants are appropriate in addition to your breast lift requires candid discussion with your plastic surgeon. Make certain he or she understands your concerns, and thoroughly discusses all the options with you. Together, you can determine if implants will help you to achieve your goals.

Read Part 4 about breast implants and Part 8 about breast augmentation if you are considering increasing the size of your breasts, or if your pla stic surgeon recommends breast implants in addition to your breast lift.

PART TEN

Other Breast Surgery Procedures

Are any breast surgeries commonly performed together?

What other plastic surgery procedures are commonly performed with breast surgery?

How are disproportionate breasts corrected?

More ...

84. Are any breast surgeries commonly performed together?

Every breast procedure can be performed in combination with another. Breast lift and breast augmentation are commonly performed together. Breast lift and breast reduction are very similar in techniques, and often a lift includes a minor reduction in breast volume. In nearly every case of breast reconstruction, a breast lift, reduction, or augmentation may be performed on the opposite breast to achieve symmetry. Ironically, even a reduction on one breast and an augmentation on the other can be performed together, if the goal is to correct severe disproportion between the breasts.

85. What other plastic surgery procedures are commonly performed with breast surgery?

The important word here is "commonly," because common or not, any breast surgery theoretically could be performed at the same surgical session as any other plastic surgery procedure. However, not all combinations of procedures in one surgical setting are most appropriate nor are they in your best interests.

Common plastic surgery procedures performed in conjunction with breast surgery include:

- Tummy tuck
- Limited liposuction
- Surgical body lifts

This doesn't mean that a facelift, rhinoplasty, or other facial procedures cannot be safely performed at the same time as breast surgery, but it does make sense to plan similar procedures together. This can benefit your safety in the duration of anesthesia as well as other factors such as fluid and blood loss. Having like procedures performed together can benefit your recovery. It makes sense to be focused on only one general region of healing at a time.

86. How are disproportionate breasts corrected?

Disproportionate breasts are corrected by a combination of plastic surgery procedures that will correct differences between the breasts, and result in breasts that are proportionate to your body. For example, if one breast is overly large and the other has no normal breast development, your plastic surgeon will likely reduce the large breast and augment the breast with no normal growth, or reconstruct it using techniques similar to post-mastectomy reconstruction. The result will be proportion between the breasts and to your body. Or, if one breast is of normal size and the second overly large, your plastic surgeon may reduce one breast and perform a minor lift on the second, so that the breasts match in size, shape, and position.

Just as the overall size, shape, and position of women's breasts varies greatly, so too does the disproportion women experience between their breasts. Therefore, your best option in having your disproportionate breasts corrected is to have a thorough consultation and examination with a board-certified plastic surgeon who is experienced in all facets of breast surgery. Discuss your goals and what you hope your final outcomes to be, and consider how your breasts may continue to change based on your age and future growth, and such things as future pregnancies. Only then can you and your plastic surgeon agree on the best approach to correcting your breast asymmetry and helping you to achieve your goals.

While correction of severe breast disproportion is considered reconstructive, not all insurers will cover your surgery, and some have specific standards of how they define a disfigurement significant enough for reimbursement. Your best approach to insurance coverage is to first, have a thorough examination, report, and referral to a plastic surgeon documented by your gynecologist or primary care provider, and submit it to your insurer. Then, your plastic surgeon will need to complete paperwork that may include the submission of photographs of your condition to your insurer in order to receive precertification. However, even if you have followed all of the necessary protocols for coverage, don't believe that your insurance will cover any portion of your procedure unless you have pre-certification in writing.

87. What other forms of breast surgery are performed?

Breast surgery can also be performed to treat breast anomalies or unexpected conditions that are not readily classified. Breast anomalies may be **congenital** (present at birth) or acquired. Acquired anomalies include such things as **trauma** or injury to the breast.

A significant blow to the breast or any other physical force can result in ruptured blood vessels that may cause localized bleeding, called a *hematoma*. The hematoma can be felt as a lump and may need to be

Congenital
present at birth.

Trauma
a physical or mental injury.

surgically drained. In addition, trauma to the breast can damage delicate breast tissue, mammary glands, and fat cells. This can result in a condition called necrosis, where the injured tissue forms a hard lump. While such a lump is not cancerous, it may need to be removed, and depending on the size and location of the necrosis, you may require reconstruction.

Other forms of trauma range from a nipple piercing that becomes infected to wounds acquired from accidents and acts of violence. If surgery is a prescribed course of treatment, it is considered reconstructive. However, pre-certification, if possible, is recommended. If trauma to your breasts is the result of an act of violence, surgery can correct your disfigurement. But equally important to restoring your breast is that action is taken against the person who inflicted your injuries, for your protection and the protection of all women. Surgery to treat trauma and restore your breast can give you new hope and confidence, and your best chance at feeling confident in yourself will come from breast surgery and victim counseling.

Congenital anomalies vary, as do the procedures to treat these conditions. Breast surgery to treat congenital anomalies is a highly specialized segment of breast surgery. Make certain the plastic surgeon you choose has training *and* experience in treating congenital breast anomalies.

88. What congenital deformities are addressed by breast surgery?

Congenital deformities treated by breast surgery generally correct deformed or irregular breast development or a complete lack of development in one or both breasts. Deformities to the appearance of the breast include breast size and shape, the absence of a normal nipple and areola, or presence of more than one nipple. The techniques used to treat congenital deformities depend on the deformities themselves and the resulting conditions.

Specific conditions treated by breast reconstruction techniques include:

- **Amastia:** a rare condition where normal growth of the breast or nipple and areola does not occur. This can be present in one or both breasts, and is often related to other birth defects.
- **Amazia:** the absence of a nipple and areola.
- **Asymmetry:** where the breasts develop at a significant disproportion.
- **Axillary breasts:** where breast tissue develops or is located in the underarm region. Flap techniques can reposition the tissue to a more natural position on the chest wall.
- **Chest wall abnormalities:** where deformities in the chest wall that result from other congenital conditions or even developmental disorders such as severe scoliosis, affect normal breast development and appearance.
- **Poland syndrome:** the symptoms include a lack of a portion of the pectoralis (chest wall) muscle that may contribute to the lack of breast development.

Any of the above conditions should first be diagnosed by your primary care physician or a pediatric specialist. Diagnostic tests to verify the conditions and any underlying contributing causes will likely be required. A consultation with a plastic surgeon can begin at any age, to monitor progress and development, and define an appropriate course and timing for treatment.

Amastia

a rare condition where normal growth of the breast or nipple and areola does not occur; can be present in one or both breasts, and is often related to other birth defects.

Amazia

the absence of a nipple and areola.

Asymmetric breasts

the breasts develop at a significant disproportion in size or shape.

Axillary breasts

where breast tissue develops or is located in the underarm region; flap techniques can reposition the tissue to a more natural position on the chest wall.

Poland syndrome

a disorder where there is a lack of a portion of the pectoralis (chest wall) muscle, which may contribute to the lack of breast development.

Other congenital breast deformities treated by specific breast surgery procedures include:

- **Breast or juvenile hypertrophy:** where the breast growth is in excess beyond the normal stages of growth in life; can be treated by breast reduction (see Part 7).
- **Constricted breasts:** where the breasts fold is high, and breast tissue is constricted to the upper portion of the breast (see Part 8).
- **Tubular breasts:** where the breasts have no natural slope or roundness, but rather appear as tubes projecting out from the chest wall (the placement of breast implants and/or breast lift can change them to a more natural appearance (see Parts 8 and 9).
- **Ptosis:** severe flattening and dropping of the breasts (see Question 80).

Congenital Deformities

Nearly every congenital breast deformity can be addressed by reconstruction. The greater issues for defining good candidates of reconstruction due to congenital deformities are:

- Health factors related or not to the breast deformity
- The exact type of deformity and structures of the breast and body afflicted
- Timing and physical development of the patient

In general, good candidates for breast surgery to correct congenital deformities are young women whose physical growth is nearing completion (around age 16 years). However, where only limited structures of the breast are involved (such as the nipple and areola), or where good candidates understand that reconstruction may evolve over several procedures and time, recon-

Other Breast Surgery Procedures

Breast or juvenile hypertrophy
where the breast growth is in excess beyond the normal stages of growth in life; can be treated by breast reduction.

Constricted breasts
where the breast fold is high and breast tissue is constricted to the upper portion of the breast.

Tubular breasts
where the breasts have no natural slope or roundness, but rather appear as tubes projecting out from the chest wall.

struction may begin at any age defined as appropriate by your plastic surgeon. Multiple procedures are not necessarily required to correct a deformity, but rather to address the deformity according to the various stages at which a woman's body matures, or refine initial outcomes that may change somewhat as a woman grows and matures.

PART ELEVEN

Following Breast Surgery

When will I see the results of my breast surgery?

How long is recovery following breast surgery?

How should I care for my breasts following breast surgery?

More ...

89. When will I see the results of my breast surgery?

Nearly every breast surgery, except for reconstruction techniques using tissue expansion, result in immediate and visible changes to a woman's breasts. However, post-surgical swelling and other conditions require time to resolve. Given the soft nature of breast tissue, your breasts will settle a bit over time, resulting in their final appearance anywhere from a few weeks to a few months following surgery.

In addition, just as any part of your body changes through time, aging, and with weight fluctuations, so too will your breasts. Therefore, while nearly all breast surgery is permanent, the appearance of your breasts will change over time.

90. How long is recovery following breast surgery?

Recovery following breast surgery is variable based on a number of things.

- The procedure or procedures you will have
- The extent of the procedure(s)
- Your overall health
- The anesthesia used
- Any other procedures performed in conjunction with your breast surgery
- Your own personal determination to get back to your regular routine

A discussion of the recovery process relative to the specific breast surgery procedures discussed in this book is included with each procedure. This includes general information of how long your recovery is expected to take, what you will experience during your recovery, and your obligations as a patient.

The specifics of *your* recovery are part of the informed consent process you will undergo prior to consenting to surgery. If you have any questions at all, ask them directly to your plastic surgeon and his or her staff, and keep asking questions until you get answers you understand.

You must, however, accept and exhibit patience. There are trade-offs to quick recoveries and those are likely to affect outcomes and risks to your health. Therefore, follow all of the instructions you are given and accept the various stages of recovery you will experience. When in recovery, returning to a normal daily routine seems very far away. But once you do return to your normal daily routine, the time invested in your recovery will be a small investment and a brief memory, necessary to achieve your goals.

91. How should I care for my breasts following breast surgery?

Each procedure has specific considerations for post-operative care that are included with each breast surgery procedure discussed in this book. How you specifically should care for your breasts will be defined by your plastic surgeon in the informed consent process.

In general, regardless of the breast surgery procedure you will have, it is important to do a few things.

- Follow all wound care instructions specifically, including changing dressings; cleansing; and application of creams, ointments, gels, or tape. This will

help prevent infection of the incisions and the formation of irregular or excessive scars.

- Follow all instructions for wearing support garments specifically. Once your recovery is complete,
regularly and consistently wear bras or clothing with
appropriately sized and comfortable breast support.
- Protect your breasts from injury by wearing proper
support during exercise.
- Practice regular self-breast exams and have regular
breast exams including mammograms or other
screenings in the frequency and manner defined by
your breast surgeon or plastic surgeon, and your
personal physician.

While it is important to properly care for your breasts,
having breast surgery will not limit your physical ability once you have recovered. Therefore, don't use breast
surgery as an excuse not to do the things that you
know you can do. The potential for serious injury
comes from truly pushing your limits or from accidents, not from normal and accepted physical activity.

92. What are possible complications following breast surgery?

Breast surgery carries the same risks as any surgical
procedure. These are discussed thoroughly in Question
19 and include: poor healing of incisions, bleeding,
infection, pulmonary emboli, anesthesia complications,
and unexpected complications related to individual
procedures. The potential to develop these complications following breast surgery is related to your overall
health and the extent of your procedure. They cannot
in any way be fully predicted.

Additional complications include a temporary or permanent loss of sensation in the breast or nipple, asymmetry, and risks related to each procedure specifically. For example, the use of breast implants has the added risk of capsular contracture, and implant rupture, leaking, or deflation.

Therefore, to minimize your risk of any complication, follow all of the instructions you are given, to the letter. If you slip—for example, you take an aspirin or have a cigarette when instructed not to—make certain to tell your plastic surgeon right away. For your safety, your surgery may need to be postponed. Waiting an extra week or more to undergo surgery is certainly a fair trade-off to avoiding what has been scientifically proven to increase the potential for complications. If you fail to follow instructions that you are given after surgery, tell your plastic surgeon right away. You and your plastic surgeon will need to evaluate your condition, perhaps revise your instructions, and review all of your instructions once again, so that you understand and accept that the imperative for good results and good healing requires your cooperation.

Scars are not a risk of breast surgery; they are to be expected. However, how you heal and the formation of irregular scars is a risk that can often be carefully controlled. This is very much in your control and requires following all of the instructions that you are given regarding wound care and healing. Also, a breast that does not fully appear or feel completely natural is not a risk of breast surgery. This is one of the trade-offs you must consider when electing some breast surgery procedures.

93. Can pain be controlled?

The reality of any surgery is that you will experience some discomfort. Your surgeon should be candid with you about the pain that you are likely to experience and discuss the various means to control that pain. You need to directly share your ability to cope with pain and your pain thresholds with your surgeon. Pain management is an important part of breast surgery, and your surgeon will provide you a means to cope. However, it is equally important during the recovery process to surround yourself with people and things that comfort you. Place yourself in an environment of serenity and put aside anything (or anyone) that causes you stress.

There are many means of controlling pain. Today, prescription or over-the-counter oral pain medications work safely and well to lessen moderate pain. For individuals who cannot tolerate these medications and who don't like some of the associated side effects such as nausea or drowsiness, there is an alternative that is now commonly used following surgery: a pain pump. A **pain pump** is small handheld device attached to thin tubing that leads to your incision or surgical site. The pain pump delivers local anesthetic to the surgical site only, thereby lessening your discomfort and the side effects of pain medications. The advantages are that only the surgical site is treated, and that you have control of your pain. However, pain pumps are only temporary. You must accept a little discomfort during the recovery process.

Acute pain, or a sudden onset of new pain is not something you must accept, however. If this is something you experience, contact your surgeon right away.

Pain pump

a small handheld device attached to thin tubing that leads to an incision or surgical site used to temporarily deliver a local anesthetic to the surgical site only; discomfort is reduced and there are fewer side effects than with pain medications.

94. How can I camouflage the signs that I have had surgery?

When clothed, no one will likely notice you have had breast surgery, even in the first few days following surgery. During that time, if you are swollen and sore, loose, comfortable clothing that buttons or zips in front is your best bet. You won't want to be pulling anything over your head in those first few days after any kind of breast surgery. Once you are out and about, a shirt or sweater that fits you properly, even one that is more fitted, will easily conceal a support bra or any swelling.

Set aside or purchase a few support bras and tops in varying styles prior to your surgery. Cotton bras are generally more comfortable during healing, as is a front closure. Make certain you don't wear bras or support garments with underwires until you are advised that you may wear them. During the first few weeks after breast surgery, before your breast position and shape fully settle, don't wear anything too revealing. When you follow these measures, it is likely your breast surgery won't be revealed.

When you are ready to wear a swimsuit, one that is more athletic in design or that is designed with a built-in shelf bra will likely be more comfortable, more flattering, and provide more coverage. But once you have healed completely and breast position has settled, any swimsuit or clothing that makes *you* feel comfortable and confident is your limit.

PART TWELVE

Your Future

Can breast surgery procedures be repeated?

Will I always have visible scars from breast surgery?

What if I am not pleased with the outcome
of my breast surgery?

More ...

95. Can breast surgery procedures be repeated?

A woman's body, her life, and her personal preferences change over time. These reasons alone are why many women undergo breast surgery more than once: to further reduce a prior reduction, to re-lift an aging breast lift, to refine a breast reconstruction, or to enlarge or refresh a prior augmentation. In some cases, many years may pass before a procedure is repeated. In other cases, only months may pass before a woman needs to, or decides to have additional breast surgery.

In the case of breast implants, you must accept that placement of breast implants can and likely will be repeated during the course of a woman's life. At present, no breast implant is approved by the U.S. FDA to be a lifetime device. Despite that it is highly durable and impact-proof, implants may rupture, leak, and deflate. Over time they don't necessarily change with a woman's body. Therefore, if you have breast implants, not only can they be replaced, they likely will need to be replaced.

96. Will I always have visible scars from breast surgery?

Plastic surgery of the breast can create very natural results in nearly every case. But to achieve those results, there are trade-offs, namely the appearance of scars. Surgery cannot be performed without **incisions**, and every incision will leave some visible mark on the skin. Modern techniques limit the size of scars and allow for incision placement in inconspicuous places, and advances in wound healing can minimize the irregular appearance of scars. But regardless, every plastic sur-

Incision

a cut; surgical wound; a division of soft tissue, usually by a knife.

gery procedure of the breast today requires an incision of some kind that will leave a scar, somewhere.

I have always looked upon scars as reminders of events in life. Those events may have been painful or unpleasant, but scars represent that healing is complete; that there is closure to the pain and unpleasantness. You need to decide if what you feel about your breasts is worth the trade-off of any scars that result. I know my scars remind me to put breast cancer behind me.

—Ann

I wasn't putting disease behind me, but a lot of physical and emotional stress. I agree with Ann: you need to decide if the trade-off of resulting scars are worth your true end result and how that result will affect your self-image, your confidence, and your life.

—Lauren

97. What if I am not pleased with the outcome of my breast surgery?

First, define why you are not pleased. Base your definition on the realistic goals for your breast surgery discussed and agreed upon with your plastic surgeon prior to the surgery. Then discuss your dissatisfaction with your plastic surgeon. Among the considerations to discuss are:

- Whether or not your outcomes are final
- What specifically in your goals was not met
- If the potential for your present result was something discussed with you prior to surgery
- What can be done to achieve your goals

If you took the time to choose an appropriately trained, certified, and experienced provider with whom you felt confident and comfortable, then there should be no discomfort in discussing why you are not pleased. If you feel you are not getting answers you are comfortable with or wish to seek additional advice, do so. Consult with a like provider and focus on exactly the questions above. But don't expect that provider to tell you something went wrong. He or she should focus on defining what can be done to help you meet your goals, if in fact you can achieve the outcomes you desire.

98. How can I maintain the healthy contours of my breasts following breast surgery?

Until we are able to literally stop the aging process and effects of gravity, breast contours, like any part of the body, will age and change. Maintaining healthy breast contours requires maintaining breast health, overall. This means leading a healthy lifestyle of appropriate exercise and a nutritious diet, and maintaining a stable weight. It also means caring for your breasts and breast skin properly. Wear proper breast support relative to your level of activity at all times. Care for your breast skin in the same manner you care for the skin on your face or anywhere on your body. Finally, don't forget to wear sunscreen on delicate cleavage!

Equally as important for every woman, regardless of breast health or condition, is a monthly breast self-exam, regular breast exams by your primary physician, regular follow-ups as defined by your plastic surgeon, and appropriate diagnostic testing as prescribed.

99. Will breast surgery affect my ability to breast-feed, or breast sensation?

Your ability to breast-feed after breast surgery depends on a number of factors:

- The type of breast surgery
- How it affected your mammary (milk producing) glands
- How it affected your nipple
- Your own determination

You will never be able to breast-feed naturally from a reconstructed breast. Following breast reduction, breast lift, or breast augmentation, your ability to breast-feed is variable.

There are devices that have been developed specifically for mothers who cannot naturally breast-feed that still give your child the experience of nursing. If your future ability to breast-feed is an important issue to you, discuss this with your surgeon prior to surgery. It may be in your best interests to postpone surgery, if the guarantee of breast-feeding naturally is more important to you than your goals for breast surgery.

Much like the ability to breast-feed, breast sensation is highly variable following breast surgery. A reconstructed breast will never have the same sensation as a natural breast. However, that does not mean that you will be without sensation entirely. Over time and with your own determination, you may experience limited breast sensation.

There is no way to predict what you personally will experience with regard to breast sensation following surgery. Nor is it possible to predict if you will experience anything different in sensation at all. If you have had a breast reduction or lift, and the nipple has been repositioned, you may lose some of your natural sensation, or it may be heightened. With a breast augmentation, the placement of the implant and pressure it has on breast tissue and nerves can either lessen or heighten nipple sensation.

100. How will having breast surgery affect my life?

Breast surgery is an amazingly positive experience for the hundreds of thousands of women who undergo procedures each year. It can give a woman newfound confidence in her body and in herself. But, like any surgical experience, it includes anxiety, stress, wonder, discomfort, healing, and the excitement of goals realized.

The effects of breast surgery are as positive and rewarding as you wish them to be. If you choose to have breast surgery, you will likely find that you are not just a statistic among all women who undergo breast surgery procedures. In addition, you will find that you are among the millions of women who over their lifetime experience the fulfillment of your own initiative to make your goals for your breasts, and for your life, happen.

Breast surgery affected my life. It made me feel confident about my body and my appearance. But you don't spend every day of the rest of your life thinking about your breast implants or surgery. It just becomes a part of who you are.

—Kristin

Afterword

In the last decades of the 20th century and in these first few years of the 21st century, there have been major medical advances of all kinds. There is no question that the pace of the research and development necessary for treatment and surgical innovation will continue. For women in advanced societies, the innovations of the future include preserving women's health and improvements in women's options for both elective and medically necessary breast surgery. These innovations will include, in some cases, a blurring of lines between elective and medically necessary breast surgery.

Onco-plastics is a term you may be hearing more about in the very near future. Its focus is twofold: to treat breast cancer (oncology) and to restore the breast appearance (plastic surgery) through one concerted view of a team of medical specialists. Today, while the law allows women the right to reconstruction, the information and the initiative to restore a woman to feel whole again is not always easy to access. Onco-plastics will become the standard to address reconstruction at the time of recommending treatment, and incorporating reconstruction goals into the prescribed treatment.

Onco-plastics
a term describing surgeons trained in treating breast cancer (oncology) and restoring the breast appearance (plastic surgery) through one concerted view of a team of specialists.

Breast reduction in the perspective of the insurer has always been fuzzy when it comes to determining whether it is elective or medically necessary. But the health-preserving and cancer-prevention benefits of breast reduction will likely continue to be aggressively researched and reported. Hopefully, this will lead to a mandate of insurance coverage for the millions of women whose quality of life is impaired by overly large breasts and/or whose breast cancer risk may be elevated.

Your Future

Much like in the case of breast reconstruction, the advances in surgical techniques for breast reduction must not be held back because of low reimbursement from insurers. Shorter incisions, smaller resulting scars, more natural outcomes, less risk, and improved recovery experiences must continue to advance for breast reconstruction, breast reduction, and elective breast surgeries.

The greatest advancement we will likely see among all breast surgeries is in the breast implant, both for reconstruction and augmentation. Whether the new generation of silicone implants proves to be an optimal solution, or newer substances of more viscous fillers such as polyethylene glycol and saline, or hyaluronic acid become the standard in safe, naturally feeling and looking implants is something that only time will tell. In fact, there may be even more filler substances we begin to hear of in the future as well as new implant coatings. Titanium, the most biocompatible of non-porous substances, is being tested in a microthin coating for breast implants, with the hope of eliminating the potential for rupture, leakage, sweating, or bleeding of any breast implant.

The one likely advancement that will not be positive in the realm of breast surgery is the constantly advancing social debate of the value of breast surgery, and biased media coverage of it. The bottom line is that educated women, with appropriately trained physicians, the proper personal support, and education to make confident choices can and should act in a manner that is personally best. No women's rights organization should tell a woman what to do. No educated woman should be influenced by biased messages. Media should report all the facts, and not bias or sensationalize the value of education. Women should read between the lines and most importantly always look to scientifically valid sources for information such as the two recognized medical specialty organizations in plastic surgery: the American Society of Plastic Surgeons and the American Society for Aesthetic Plastic Surgery.

Most importantly, every woman must do what is right for her confidence, her body, and her life. No woman must let anyone dictate to her; however, she should have a skilled physician and the support of family and friends in making that decision.

If breast surgery were not the healthy, fulfilling choice or treatment that it is, it would not be advancing. Medical science would look for other ways. But in view of the growing number of breast surgeries every year, in every category except breast reconstruction, one thing about breast surgery is clear: The results of elective and medically necessary breast surgery are continuously improving in aesthetic results and achieving the personal satisfaction of well over one million women who undergo breast surgery every year.

It is your choice. Ask questions, question answers, and make the confident choice that is right for you, today and for your future.

Glossary

Ablative breast surgery: A type of surgery to remove all or part of the breast.

Accreditation: A hospital, outpatient setting, or ambulatory surgical facility that has passed national and/or state regulated requirements for architecture, medical equipment, procedural protocols, and then inspection; must also adhere to all local, state, and national regulations including sanitation, fire safety, and building codes.

Aesthetic plastic surgery of the breast: Procedures elected strictly to improve breast appearance and a woman's appearance overall.

Amastia: A rare condition where normal growth of the breast or nipple and areola does not occur; can be present in one or both breasts, and is often related to other birth defects.

Amazia: The absence of a nipple and areola.

Anesthesia: Loss of physical sensation resulting from pharmacologic depression of nerve function or from neurologic dysfunction; broad term for anesthesiology as a clinical specialty.

Anesthesiologist: A physician specializing solely in anesthesiology and related areas, who is board certified and legally qualified to administer anesthetics and related techniques.

Areola: The dark tissue surrounding the nipple of the breast.

Aspiration: Removal of fluid collected inside a body cavity with a needle.

Asymmetric breasts: The breasts develop at a significant disproportion in size or shape.

Augmentation mammaplasty: A breast augmentation to enhance the size of the breast by surgically placing an implant in the breast.

Axilla: The underarm area.

Axillary breasts: A condition where breast tissue develops or is located in the underarm region; flap techniques can reposition the tissue to a more natural position on the chest wall.

Baker scale: A standardized test to measure capsular contracture varying from Grade I (breast is normally soft and natural appearing) to Grade IV (breast is very firm, with clearly visible distortion in shape, and the patient may experience pain).

Benign: A non-malignant neoplasm or mild character of an illness.

Bilateral mastectomy: Surgical removal of both breasts.

Board certification: A process following the completion of medical school that includes several years of additional training in a medical specialty, written and oral exams, and continuing hours of education after certification by a nationally and internationally recognized organization.

Body dysmorphic disorder (BDD): A psychosomatic (an influence of the mind over the body) characterized by a preoccupation with some imagined defect in appearance in a normal-appearing person.

BRCA1 and *BRCA2:* Genes found to be linked to a predisposition for breast cancer.

Breast augmentation: Procedure to make small breasts larger.

Breast conserving surgery: Lumpectomy is followed by radiation; considered an alternative in some cases for a masectomy.

Breast implants: Medical devices that are surgically implanted into a woman's body to: (1) enhance and enlarge breast size and shape in breast augmentation; (2) create the substance of a breast mound for breast reconstruction following mastectomy or other surgery to treat breast cancer; (3) restore a more normal appearance to a woman's body that is lacking a breast due to congenital anomaly or birth defect.

Breast lift: Procedure to restore the appearance of a sagging, flat breast.

Breast or juvenile hypertrophy: Where the breast growth is in excess beyond the normal stages of growth in life; can be treated by breast reduction.

Breast reconstruction: A type of surgery to restore the physical appearance of a breast resulting most often from acquired deformities. Acquired deformities are those where a breast has been completely lost or disfigured as the result of breast surgery to treat breast disease or trauma.

Breast reduction: A type of surgery that removes fat and/or glandular tissue to reduce size and reshape a woman's breasts.

Breast surgery: Any medical procedure that penetrates beyond the surface of breast skin. Includes: (1) procedures to diagnose and treat breast disease including cancer and benign cysts, tumors, and growths; (2) procedures to change the appearance of a breast, including restoring the absence of a breast, increase or decrease in breast size, or revision of breast shape and position; and (3) surgery to prevent breast disease.

Calcification: A condition where calcium deposits develop around the breast implant capsule, causing firmness and occasionally pain.

Capsular contracture: Excess scar tissue constricts over time; may occur with breast implants.

CBC: Complete blood count. Using a volume of a millimeter of blood, the number of red blood cells (RBCs), white blood cells (WBCs), erythrocyte indices, hematocrit, differential blood count, and sometimes the platelet count are calculated.

Certified registered nurse anesthetist (CRNA): A registered professional nurse with additional education and certification in the administration of anesthetics.

Clear margin: Area around a tumor that shows no preliminary evidence of cancerous cells.

Closed capsulotomy: A controversial technique that is not recommended to treat capsular contracture; involves a very forceful squeezing of the breast capsule to release or tear it; can result in implant rupture and localized bleeding, and may void the breast implant manufacturer's warranty.

Congenital: Present at birth.

Constricted breasts: Where the breast fold is high and breast tissue is constricted to the upper portion of the breast.

DIEP (deep inferior epigastric perforator) flap: Type of free flap breast reconstruction where a flap of skin and fat are taken from the abdomen; however, does not include the rectus muscle.

Drains: Medical tubing placed in wound cavities to remove fluid.

Electrocardiogram (ECG): A graphic record of the heart's integrated action currents obtained with the electrocardiograph displayed as voltage changes over time.

Endoscope: A type of microsurgical instrument that is basically a hollow tube; an implant can be placed in the breast and then filled using this tool.

Excised: Fat, tissue, and glands are separated from the surrounding tissues and removed.

External prosthesis: A non-surgical alternative after breast surgery, that is a padded, artificial breast that is held in place by an undergarment.

Extrusion: Where a breast implant actually breaks through to the skin surface and becomes exposed.

Free flap: A type of breast reconstruction that uses a woman's own muscle, fat, and skin from the abdomen, buttocks, or thigh, transplanted to the chest wall, using microsurgical techniques.

Free TRAM (transverse rectus abdominus musculocutaneous) flap: Type of free flap breast reconstruction where a flap of skin, fat, and sometimes muscle are taken from the abdomen like a pedicled TRAM, but are completely detached from the abdomen; used to reform the breast.

GAP (gluteal artery perforator) flap: Type of free flap breast reconstruction where skin and fat are taken from the gluteus or buttocks, from the superior gluteal (S-GAP) or inferior gluteal (I-GAP) regions.

General breast surgery: To diagnose and treat breast disease through the removal of the entire breast, or only of diseased tissue, tumors, or cysts.

Granulomas: Nodular inflammatory lesions, usually small or granular, firm, persistent, and containing compactly grouped cells.

Gynecomastia: Excessive development of male mammary glands.

Hematoma: Bleeding externally or under the skin.

Immediate reconstruction: Breast reconstruction performed at the time of mastectomy.

Incision: A cut; surgical wound; a division of soft tissue, usually by a knife.

Infection: Invasion of the body with organisms that have the potential to cause disease.

Informed consent: The process a patient is taken through that defines a procedure prescribed to treat a condition, the risks and potential outcomes of the procedure, and a patient's potential alternatives.

In situ breast cancer: When cancer cells are contained within the milk ducts.

Intravenous (IV): Within a vein or veins.

Invasive breast cancer: When cancer cells migrate to tissues outside of the confines of the milk ducts.

Latissimus dorsi flap: A type of reconstruction surgery using a woman's own muscle, fat, and skin from her back; most often used to support a breast implant where little tissue remains at the chest wall to support and cover the implant. In a minor percentage of cases, this flap alone may be used to reconstruct the breast.

Lumpectomy: Type of surgical removal of a tumor involving breast conserving surgery.

Macromastia: A condition characterized by overly large, pendulous breasts.

Magnetic resonance imaging (MRI): A type of diagnostic radiologic technique using nuclear magnetic resonance technology to provide three-dimensional pictures from inside a body to check for health and disease.

Mammogram: A graphic record produced by mammography, which is a radiologic examination of the female breast with equipment and techniques designed to screen for cancer.

Margin: Area of healthy tissue surrounding a tumor, cyst, or calcification; surgically removed with the lump to make certain all of the abnormal tissue cells are included.

Mastectomy: Complete surgical removal of the breast, most often including the nipple/areola complex. A simple or total mastectomy includes all breast tissue, down to, but not including, the chest wall muscle or the lymph glands. The result is the complete absence of a breast on the chest wall, with a horizontal scar where the breast was once located.

Mastopexy: A breast lift surgery to raise and reshape a flat, sagging breast.

Microsurgery: The reattachment of nerves and vessels in surgery is performed via microscope and micro-sized surgical tools.

Modified radical mastectomy: A type of mastectomy that includes the removal of the axillary (underarm) lymph nodes.

Mortality: Death.

Necrosis: Death of one or more cells, or of a portion of tissue or organ, that results in permanent damage.

Negative margins: No additional malignant cells are in tissue surrounding the tumor.

Onco-plastics: A term describing surgeons trained in treating breast cancer (oncology) and restoring the breast appearance (plastic surgery) through one concerted view of a team of specialists.

Pain pump: A small handheld device attached to thin tubing that leads to an incision or surgical site used to temporarily deliver a local anesthetic to the surgical site only; discomfort is reduced and there are fewer side effects than with pain medications.

Palpable: Capable of being felt in an examination by the hands.

Partial or segmental mastectomy: A type of mastectomy where a larger segment of the breast than a lumpectomy is surgically removed, but some of the breast tissue and skin are pre-served, and, in limited cases, the nipple/areola complex are also preserved.

Pectoral muscle: A type of muscle located in the chest.

Pedicled TRAM: Transverse rectus abdominus musculocutaneous flap for a type of breast reconstruction; uses a woman's own muscle, fat, and skin from her abdomen; remains tethered to its original blood supply.

Perioperative: Around the time of the surgery.

Plastic surgery of the breast: Any surgical procedure that changes or restores the appearance of the breast, including those procedures to treat and prevent breast disease that result in the change of a breast appearance.

Plastic surgery for breast reconstruction: A specialty of medicine that includes board-certified training specific to the techniques and procedures that rebuild a woman's breast.

Poland syndrome: A disorder where there is a lack of a portion of the pectoralis (chest wall) muscle, which may contribute to the lack of breast development.

Preventative (or prophylactic) mastectomy: The removal of one or both breasts to prevent breast cancer from developing in a woman with a family history of breast cancer or to reduce a woman's chance of developing breast cancer.

Privileges: A type of agreement for a physician to operate in a particular accredited hospital; the doctor's credentials, knowledge, and training, medical standards in a particular specialty, and skills are rigorously examined by his or her peers before privileges are extended.

Prosthetic enhancements: Artificial parts of the body that help the figure to appear more natural; are removable.

Ptosis: Sagging, drooping, or falling down of bodily tissues or organs.

Pulmonary embolism: Blockage of a lung artery; can be fatal.

Quadrantectomy: A wide excision biopsy involving the removal of one quarter or quadrant of the breast; can be highly disfiguring.

Radical mastectomy: A type of mastectomy that is performed only in extreme cases; includes the removal of the major and minor pectoral (chest) muscles.

Reconstruction: A type of surgery to restore the breast at the time of or following mastectomy.

Reduction mammaplasty: A breast reduction to reduce the size of a large breast.

Sentinel node biopsy: Surgical procedure performed to determine if breast cancer has spread to adjoining lymph nodes.

Sequelae: The aftereffects or secondary results of a surgical procedure.

Seroma: Fluid collection in the space where tissue was removed.

SIEA (superficial inferior epigastric artery) perforator flap: Type of breast

reconstruction where skin and fat are taken from the abdomen, avoiding the rectus muscle.

Sub-glandularly placed implants: Type of implants placed on top of the chest muscle and below the breast glands.

Sub-mammary: Below the breast tissue; some implants are placed in that location.

Sub-muscular: Below the muscle; some implants are placed under the pectoral muscle.

Symmastia: A condition where the capsule or pocket in which breast implants are placed is too close, or where the breast implants displace into one large pocket, resulting in implants that meet in the middle of the chest and appear to be one big breast. Correction requires that the breast pocket be internally and permanently sutured smaller, and that implants be replaced and repositioned.

Tissue expansion: A type of reconstruction of the breast using a breast implant, where enough healthy skin and soft tissue necessary to cover an implant is not present; involves the placement of an implant that is not completely filled, or of a tissue expander (a silicone shell balloon-like device) at the breast mound. Through gradual filling of the implant or expander over many weeks, enough healthy tissue is produced to cover a breast implant.

TRAM (transverse rectus abdominus musculocutaneous): Type of breast surgery where a flap using a woman's own tissue taken from her abdomen is used to reconstruct a breast.

Trauma: A physical or mental injury.

TUBA (trans umbilical breast augmentation): A type of breast augmentation technique that uses an endoscope placed through an incision in the navel, to place and fill saline breast implants. This is highly controversial and should not be considered a routine incision site for the placement of breast implants.

Tubular breasts: The breasts have no natural slope or roundness, but rather appear as tubes projecting out from the chest wall.

Tummy tuck: Surgical procedure that removes skin and fat from the abdomen, resulting in a slimmer profile.

Index